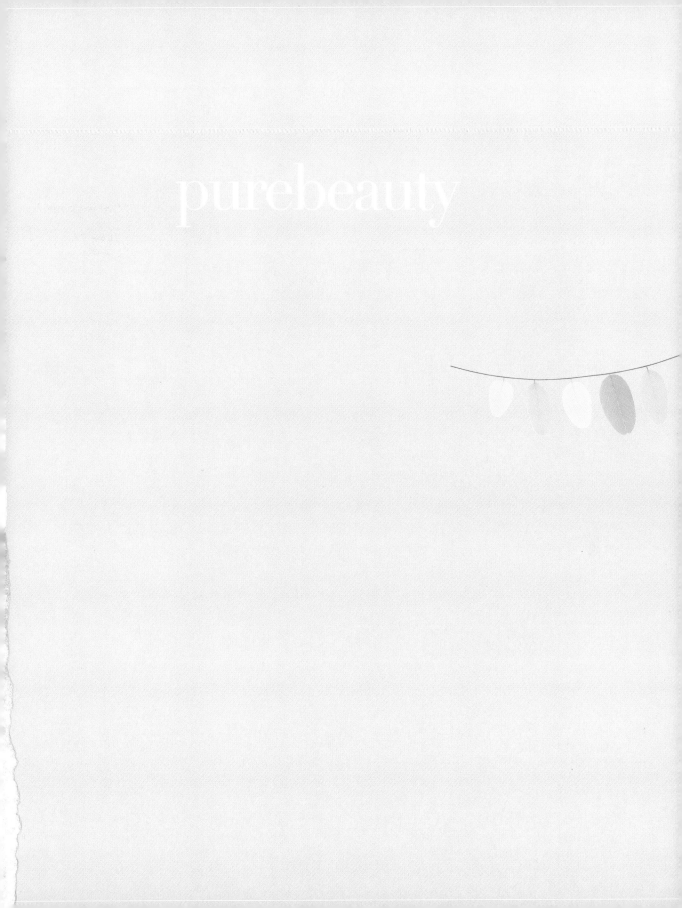

purebeauty

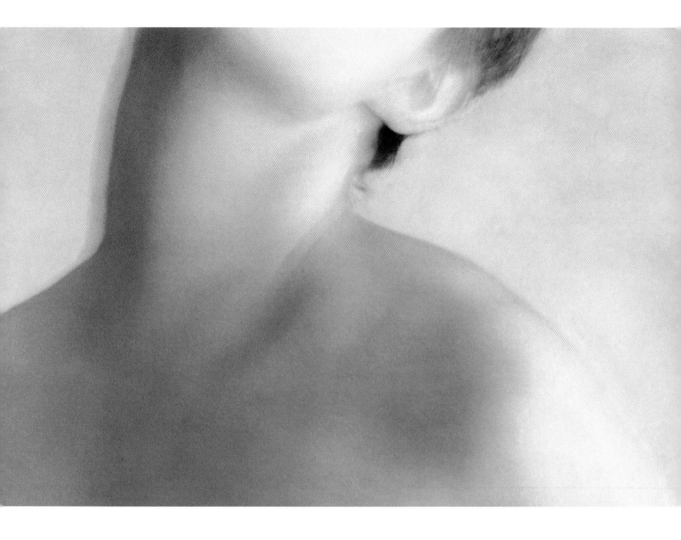

Country Living's **healthy living**

purebeauty
simple recipes for a naturally beautiful body

Mike Hulbert and Anna Carter
Foreword by Rachel Newman

Hearst Books
New York

It is the policy of William Morrow and Company, Inc., and its imprints and affiliates, recognizing the importance of preserving what has been written, to print the books we publish on acid-free paper, and we exert out best efforts to that end.

www.williammorrow.com

Library of Congress Cataloging-in-Publication Data

Hulbert, Mike, and Anna Carter

      Country living's Healthy living pure beauty / Mike Hulbert and Anna Carter.

           p. cm.

      Includes index.

      ISBN 0-688-16606-7

      1. Cosmetics.   I. Country living's Healthy living.   II Title.

TP983.H85 1999

668'.55—dc21   98-26201

                                                                                                                        CIP

Printed in Singapore

First Edition

10 9 8 7 6 5 4 3 2 1

Text set in Bauer Bodoni

Designed by Debra Sfetsios

Edited by Alanna Stang & Camilla Crichton

Produced by SMALLWOOD & STEWART, INC., New York City

contents

fore

word

Since the beginning of civilization, people
have wanted to make themselves beautiful. For
their beauty treatments they looked to Mother
Nature herself, whose goodness came naturally.
But as time passed and society changed we
all fell prey to the quick-fix promise of store-
bought cosmetics, whose contents often
contained artificial substances harmful to our
skin and to our overall health. Fortunately, the
pendulum is now swinging back, and the return
to the purity of nature is not only a desire but a
necessity. The editors of COUNTRY LIVING'S
HEALTHY LIVING are happy to bring you this
luscious collection of recipes to care naturally
for your body . . . head to toe.

Rachel Newman
Editor-in-Chief
Country Living's Healthy Living magazine

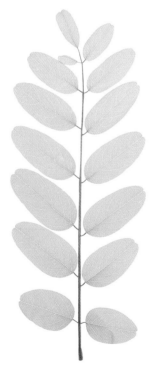

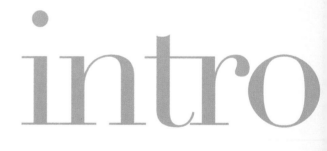

Pure beauty is glowing skin, strong nails, hair that shines right down to the roots, and an integral sense of good health and well-being radiating from your whole body.

duction

Pure Beauty is a product of a balanced lifestyle: Sound sleep, regular exercise, clean air, plenty of sunlight, and a healthful diet stimulate your entire system and help keep it toxin-free. Healthy living can put a rosy glow in your cheeks and give a sheen to your hair. It can make skin soft and supple and fingernails firm and strong.

What you choose to put on your body is as important as what you choose to put in it. When you smooth lotion onto your skin, massage shampoo through your hair, and rub conditioner into your cuticles, you are doing so in the hope that these products will beautify your appearance. But many commercial cosmetics, even some labeled "natural," may actually upset your skin's delicate hydro-lipid (water-oil) balance, clog your pores, and strip your hair and skin of their ability to naturally protect and renew themselves. Some of these products even contain fragrance chemicals that are suspected of being carcinogenic, asthma-inducing, or damaging to the respiratory, nervous, and autoimmune systems.

The all-natural beauty treatments in this book will enable you to avoid the potential perils of store-bought products. They are designed not just to lend beauty to your external appearance, but to enhance your whole being. Created from organic ingredients that naturally work with your body and your environment, they will help your skin and hair maintain an optimum balance and enable you to achieve a state of beauty you can feel right through to your core.

These recipes also invite you to experience the same simple pleasures you get from home cooking: the intangible satisfaction of creating, the meditative calm of chopping and stirring, the sensuality of working with colors and aromas, the creative pleasure of blending liquids, the fun of experimentation, and the gratification you feel when your creation is completed. You know what you have made is fresh, healthful, and untainted by chemical preservatives.

Most PURE BEAUTY recipes call for ingredients you can find in the produce or dairy section of your local market, and for utensils that are probably already in the kitchen drawer. Other recipes will ask that you familiarize yourself with items that you may be less accustomed to working with, such as essential oils and herbal or floral waters.

Before you begin to mix and measure, read all instructions and precautions. Our preparations are not complicated, but the ingredients do require proper handling and storage for best results.

Pure beauty is timeless, so it is only natural that our recipes combine ancient knowledge with modern techniques. Some of the potions derive from centuries-old treatments used in many different cultures. Others draw their strength from more recent discoveries in chemistry and botany.

Just as finding the balance between the ancient and the new is one of the joys of pure beauty, so too is the harmony achieved as we enhance our own natural beauty with the best that the organic world has to offer. As you try our recipes, we hope you will discover and treasure these same guiding principles.

Mike Hulbert and
Anna Carter

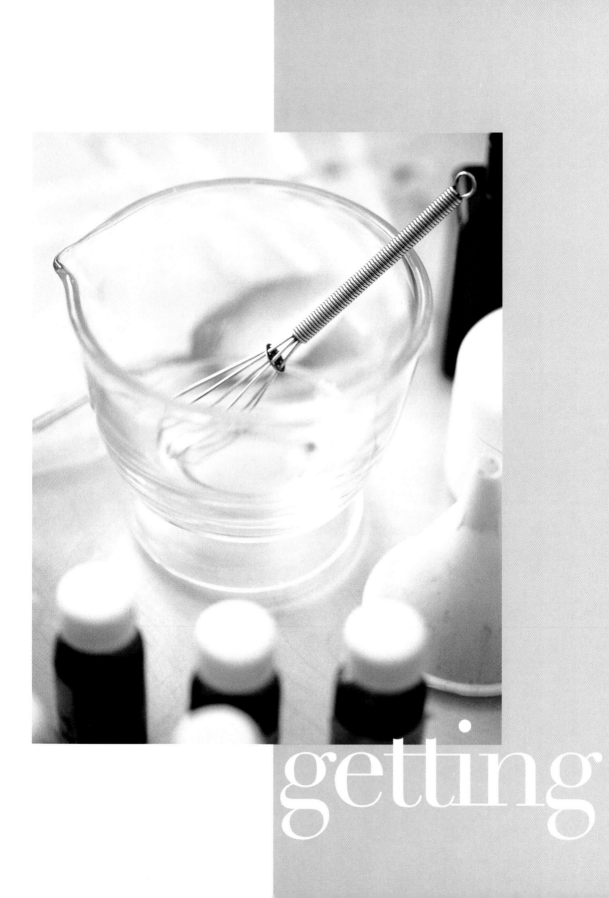

getting

Creating your own natural beauty preparations is surprisingly easy and quick. Most take only a few minutes to assemble. If you can toss together a salad, you can make cold creams and conditioners, shampoos and astringents.

Before you begin, you should, like any cook, become familiar with the ingredients, preparation techniques, precautions, and storage requirements.

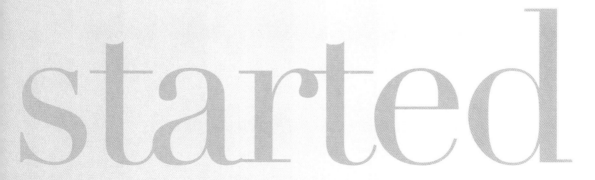
started

Ingredients

Most ingredients in our recipes fall into one of six basic groups: oils and fats, herbs, essential oils, herbal and floral waters, fruits and nuts, and dairy products. In addition, specific recipes may incorporate other ingredients such as aloe vera gel, alcohol, or beeswax.

Certain ingredients crop up again and again, in many different types of preparations. Jojoba, for example, the oil from the seed of the jojoba plant, is a jack-of-all-trades that moisturizes, softens, nourishes, tones, stimulates, and promotes healthy cell growth. Lavender is similarly multifaceted: whether it is incorporated in the form of a powdered flower, a floral water, or as an essential oil, it has a sweet, soothing scent and is antiviral, antiseptic, antifungal, and antibacterial. Glycerin appears in many recipes because it has such wide applications. It is an emollient that protects the skin and soothes inflammation, as well as a humectant that retains moisture in the skin.

Oils & Fats

Recipes for the skin often start with plant-based oils or fats derived from seeds, beans, grains, fruits, or nuts.

Like many of the natural ingredients in homemade beauty products, oils and fats do double and triple duty. The base oil determines the texture of the preparation—liquid, creamy, fluffy—so that by adding more or less to a recipe you can adjust the consistency to your preference. In addition, most oils also have therapeutic properties. They tend to be rich in essential fatty acids, substances that play a vital role in helping our skin maintain an effective barrier against the environment. As such, they make excellent moisturizers; an example is sweet almond oil, a favorite in rubbing oils and face creams. Some oils encourage healthy cell growth and others such as cold-pressed wheat germ, sunflower, and safflower oils contain vitamin E, which can speed the healing of cuts or scratches and minimize scarring.

Vegetable fats such as coconut oil, shea butter, and cocoa butter give creams a buttery consistency. They soften the skin and prevent it from drying by creating a filmy covering that traps in moisture.

Most of these oils are used in cooking and are available at better grocery or natural food markets. You may already have some of the more common oils in your pantry. If you can't find an unusual base oil called for in a recipe, you can usually substitute olive oil, which people in the olive-growing regions of the Mediterranean have relied on for many centuries to help keep their hair healthy and their skin soft and smooth.

Never substitute refined salad oils such as soy, cottonseed, or canola for the oils we recommend. These commercially prepared oils may contain high levels of preservatives or residue from pesticides or herbicides. Although the government says they are safe in food, they should be avoided for skin care.

The most desirable oils to use are cold-pressed or expeller-pressed. Cold-pressed are the least refined, but they spoil quickly, and some may have a strong, raw, earthy odor that is less desirable in certain preparations, depending on the quantity used. Expeller-pressed oils, which are produced through a chemical-free mechanical process, are somewhat more refined and last longer than cold-pressed oils. Best of all are cold-pressed organic oils, made from plants untainted by potentially harmful pesticides, fungicides, fertilizers, or herbicides.

Since oils are most effective when fresh, buy them in small quantities. Watch out for

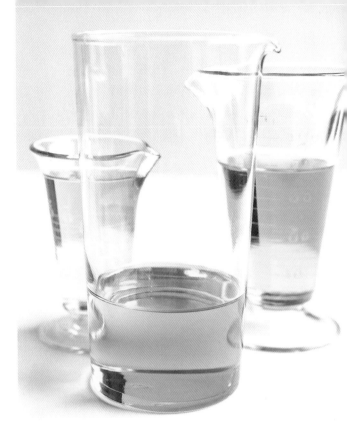

a sharp, putrid odor, which is an indication that an oil has turned rancid and should be discarded.

Herbs

If you buy herbal supplements or remedies, you may be aware that many are endowed with specific healing properties. The medicinal use of the flowers, leaves, stems, and roots of herbal plants is a broad and complex subject because almost every botanical, whether a common garden weed or a cultivated herb, has medicinal value.

A Guide to Beauty Terms

Our recipes fall into familiar categories, such as exfoliants, moisturizers, astringents, and so on. But most of our preparations work in more than one way because natural ingredients tend to have more than one beneficial quality. So a recipe for a skin softener might also cleanse and tone it; a facial might moisturize as it cleanses and exfoliates.

Astringents cause a mild inflammation of the skin tissue that improves the skin's overall appearance, making pores seem smaller so that skin looks firm and smooth. Witch hazel and floral waters are among the most common natural astringents.

Clarifying lotions are astringent and antibacterial. Like toners, they help problem skin and naturally reduce blemishes.

Emollients, such as glycerin and honey, soothe and soften the skin.

Emulsifiers, such as lecithin and beeswax, bind ingredients that have a tendency to separate, like oil and water.

Exfoliants stimulate circulation and cleanse pores by gently scrubbing the skin, ridding it of the dead cells that clog pores. Natural exfoliants, including sea salt, ground almonds, and oats, leave the skin polished and smooth.

Humectants, principally glycerin in our recipes, draw moisture to the skin from the air.

Moisturizers coat the skin, forming a seal that protects the body's natural moisture. Many natural ingredients, including wheat germ oil, jojoba, evening primrose oil, and borage oil, are natural moisturizers.

Toners help reduce blemishes by regulating and balancing sluggish and overproductive oil glands.

Historically, botany was the basis of the healing arts. It's believed that as far back as 4000 B.C., Middle Eastern kings closely guarded their stores of aloe vera, so effective was it in healing the wounds of soldiers. And in the story of the birth of Jesus Christ, the wise men are said to have brought gifts of frankincense and myrrh, two herbs traditionally valued for their healing properties.

It was during the eighteenth century that Western culture separated botany from the healing arts and defined it as the science of plant identification. Asian culture never made such a distinction. Now we find a more holistic or Eastern approach emerging in the West, as herbal treatments that were previously rejected as primitive are reintegrated into general health and beauty care practices.

The healing properties that make herbs medicinally valuable can be harnessed to improve our appearance. Naturally astringent plants gently tone and tighten skin; herbs with exfoliating properties cleanse and stimulate pores.

Certain herbs will benefit some people more than others. As you try different varieties you'll discover which are most effective for you.

Unless otherwise noted, fresh-cut herbs work best in these recipes—the fresher the better. But if you can't find fresh, you can substitute the same proportion of dried herbs, or mix fresh with dried. While flavor is more concentrated in dried herbs than in fresh, the medicinal values are approximately the same.

Gather herbs when they're in season so that you can dry and store them. Tie clean sprigs of herbs in small bunches and hang them upside down in a dry, cool, and fairly dark place with plenty of air circulation. Once their color has faded and they have turned crumbly, store them in airtight containers such as resealable plastic bags or glass jars.

Before measuring fresh herbs for recipes, they should be coarsely chopped with a knife, and dried herbs roughly crumbled. To make powdered herbs, pass dried herbs through a small herb mill or coffee grinder.

Essential Oils

Extracted from flowers, fruits, trees, and herbs, highly concentrated essential oils are natural chemical substances believed to have medicinal or therapeutic properties. While most essential oils are volatile and evaporate quickly when exposed to air, they will remain aromatically potent as molecules in the air.

The aromas of essential oils are also believed to have therapeutic properties. The science of aromatherapy is based on the principle that an aroma can directly affect the nervous system, as molecules are absorbed into the bloodstream through the mucous membranes of the nose. In aromatherapy, every oil has its own application and quality—from lavender, which is relaxing, to ylang-ylang, which is arousing.

Some essential oils might be harmful to people with especially sensitive skin or certain medical conditions. If you are taking medication, consult your physician before using any essential oils. Be sure to read the list of essential oils to avoid in Precautions (pages 28-29) and the relevant entries in the Glossary (pages 132-139) before making any recipe. Our preparations employ essential oils to improve a variety of skin conditions through external use only. We do not recommend they be taken internally.

Herbal & Floral Waters

Herbal and floral waters, or hydrosols, are safe, gentle, and less expensive alternatives to essential oils. By-products of the steam distillation process that produces essential oils, these waters contain both minute amounts of the essential oil and the water-soluble elements of the plant that are not present in the oil. They add a lovely, light fragrance to creams and lotions; some, like rose water, also as mild astringents and softeners.

Fruits & Nuts

Many preparations call for fruits and nuts. The flesh of the avocado, for example, nourishes and conditions the skin while giving preparations a creamy texture; citrus fruit juices are astringent and will dissolve makeup and surface grime.

Look for fruit that's fresh and not overripe—the type you would eat raw. If you have access to organic fruits, all the better. If you are buying from a nonorganic source, you may want to rinse fruits and vegetables with a solution of diluted hydrogen peroxide (available at most natural food markets) that is formulated to wash off any chemical residue.

Some recipes call for ground nuts, which create the abrasive action in scrubs. Ideally you should buy raw nuts to shell and grind yourself, or buy them shelled and have them ground at the local natural food market—many have machines for their customers' use. If this is not possible, buy ground nuts at the supermarket.

Eggs & Dairy

Just as you might eat eggs and drink milk to supply your body with protein and calcium, you can nourish your skin by including dairy products in your beauty care. Among the recipes in this book, you'll find cleansers that feature milk or cream as a soothing base; a hair conditioner with yogurt, which coats the shaft and restores a proper pH (alkaline and acid) balance; and herbal bath sachets with powdered dairy products to soften skin.

We recommend whole-milk products because the fats moisturize and soften skin; you won't absorb any cholesterol by massaging cream into your face.

Other Ingredients

Anyone who has baked a cake from scratch knows that oils and fats do not mix readily with water. And, once mixed, they tend to separate. The same thing happens when

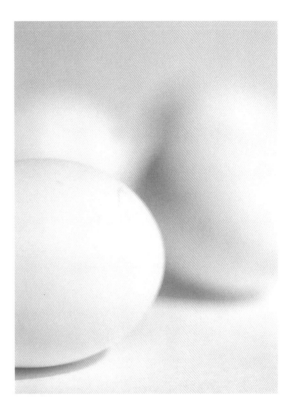

you try to mix, say, jojoba and rose water. Emulsifiers encourage oily and watery ingredients to blend and stay blended. Many synthetic beauty products use chemical emulsifiers, which can be irritating to the skin. Instead, we rely on several natural alternatives: lecithin and palm stearic acid, which are derived from vegetable oils; beeswax; borax; and emulsifying wax, which comes from botanical sources like vegetables or rice bran and is a good skin softener and cleanser.

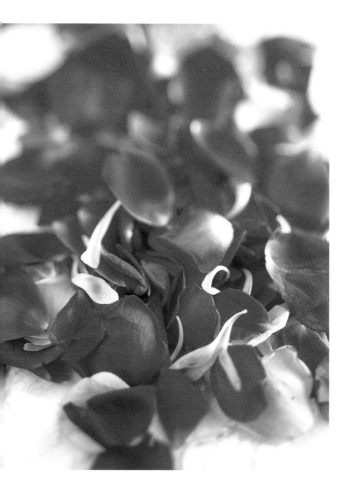

You will come across **beeswax** as a binder in recipes for lip balms, hand creams, and other skin preparations that rely on the protective barrier the wax provides against the ravages of wind and sun. Even though only a very few people are sensitive to beeswax and may suffer a slight itchy rash, be sure to test a small patch of your skin (see the instructions for skin-allergy testing in Precautions, page 29) before using beeswax in a recipe. If you do have a negative reaction, substitute a plant or vegetable wax such as wheat germ oil wax, rice bran wax, or jojoba wax, all of which are available from natural food markets and by mail order.

Honey is a wonderful emollient. It was used extensively in ancient cultures to heal wounds, and is believed to have antiseptic and antibacterial qualities. In creams and lotions it soothes the skin and leaves a micro-thin protective film.

A couple of our recipes call for **grain alcohol** because of its astringent properties. Look for the purest grain alcohol available in the liquor store; do not use the isopropyl or rubbing alcohol available in drugstores. Pure grain alcohol has no coloring or flavoring and is almost pure alcohol, which makes it superior for topical use. Some people refer to pure grain alcohol as Everclear, though this is actually a brand name. When a recipe calls for pure grain alcohol, you can substitute Everclear or vodka.

Sea salt comes in coarse, medium, and fine grades, all of which should be available in natural food markets. You can substitute coarse kosher salt from the grocery store or Epsom salts from the pharmacy.

Some of the shampoo and bath recipes include **liquid castile soap**. Because this soap base is a completely natural ingredient and doesn't contain the chemicals that create big bubbles, it may not produce much foam or lather. But it will clean as well as, if not better than, any synthetic soap. You'll find liquid castile soap in natural food markets, or you can make your own: Melt 6 cups of grated pure castile soap in a double boiler with 1 quart of distilled water. Heat the mixture, stirring gently, until the soap is dissolved. Let it cool to room temperature, then transfer it to a bottle and seal tightly. The liquid soap will keep for a year in a cool, dark place.

Equipment

Almost all the utensils you need can be found in a well-stocked kitchen.

Cookware should be made of heat-proof glass, stainless steel, or other non-porous materials.

For some of the recipes you'll need a **double boiler**, preferably made of glass, so you can see what is going on. Or you can improvise by matching a saucepan and lid with a small heat-proof mixing bowl. The bowl should sit snugly inside the saucepan with two or three inches to spare below.

A **blender** should be reserved exclusively for making these preparations.

Choose glass or glazed ceramic **mixing bowls**. Avoid bowls of unglazed pottery or anything porous, as well as bowls made of plastic or reactive metals, especially aluminum, and chipped enamelware. Essential oils can permeate plastic, and they lose their potency when they react with metal.

Use an **herb mill** or a **coffee grinder** for powdering herbs and grinding nuts and other ingredients.

Have a selection of sharp **knives** on hand for chopping and mincing.

Glass or stainless steel **measuring cups** and **spoons** will help keep proportions accurate. Avoid wooden spoons, which can splinter and retain odors.

Small rubber **spatulas** are useful for scraping mixes from bowls and for applying creams. They can be found in cosmetics and kitchen supply stores or by mail order.

Stainless steel **whisks** in a couple of

sizes will serve you well in blending solutions and preparing emulsions.

Use a fine-mesh **strainer**, unbleached paper coffee filter, or clean muslin cloth for straining your mixtures.

Glass **eye droppers** measure essential oils. Use a different dropper for each oil, but don't leave the dropper in the oil as the acids can ruin the rubber stopper. Sources for eye droppers and other special equipment are listed in Resources (pages 140-141).

Use a **funnel** to transfer completed solutions to storage bottles.

You'll need **containers** such as bottles, jars, and miscellaneous canisters for storing your preparations.

Preparation Techniques

Most of the recipes in this book are very simple to prepare—just measure and mix. None of them takes very long or involves complicated techniques. If you're looking for instant gratification, start with the masks and scrubs. Most of them can be made in a matter of minutes from items probably already in your kitchen.

Before you begin, read through the whole recipe. Assemble all the ingredients and bring them to room temperature. Protect your work area with newspaper or plastic for easy cleanup. If you set aside an ingredient or mixture as you work, cover it with a lid or a dishcloth.

Prepare the storage container so that it is ready to be filled when you finish the recipe. Make sure the bottle or jar is clean and has a tight-fitting lid. And have a funnel or spouted pitcher on hand to fill narrow-neck bottles.

Decocting & Infusing

Some recipes require making decoctions or infusions of an herb—basically, strained herbal teas. In a **decoction**, you add the herb to the water before bringing it to a boil, then turn off the heat and let the mixture steep. For an **infusion**, the herb is added to the water after it has come to a boil. We usually decoct stems, bark, roots, and twigs, but infuse the more fragile leaves and flowers.

Strain decoctions and infusions through a mesh strainer or an unbleached paper coffee filter set inside a clean funnel. You can also filter through a piece of clean fabric, and even through a clean nylon stocking, as long as it has a fine mesh so you don't end up with particles in the liquid. Always allow strained liquid to cool to room temperature before adding it to other ingredients. Steep the herb for the time indicated so that the full strength and essence of the plant's leaves, flowers, twigs, or bark are drawn into the water.

Heating Oils & Melting Waxes

To avoid the risk of ingredients burning or catching fire, always use a double boiler when heating oils and melting waxes. Fill the bottom pot with a couple inches of water, insert the top of the boiler, and add the ingredients to the top. Place the double boiler over low heat. As the water warms, its steam will melt the ingredients at an even, controlled rate. (In case of an oil fire, immediately turn off the heat and slide a lid over the pan.)

Blending Ingredients with Emulsifiers

Emulsifying — blending oily and watery ingredients with the help of a stabilizer —

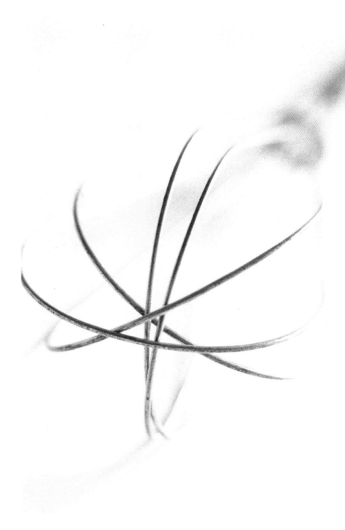

is probably the trickiest technique in making your own beauty products, but it is relatively simple to master. Begin with all the ingredients at room temperature. Heat the wax until it is just melted, then cool until it hints at turning solid. Beat in the warm oil, then add the emulsifying agent (such as borax or lecithin) and the watery ingredient to complete the emulsion. The trick is to drizzle the watery ingredient slowly at first while continually mixing the blend. (If you are not using a blender, it is a good idea to stabilize the bowl by placing it on a dampened towel.) As the water or water-based liquid incorporates and starts to blend, add it at a faster rate. Toward the end of the process, you can add the watery ingredient fairly quickly, always mixing while you pour.

Adjust the consistency of the emulsion by adding more oil for a softer feel or more melted wax to make it firmer. If you want a fluffier texture, add a small amount of the herbal or floral water (a teaspoon or less) and blend for fifteen seconds.

Yield & Use

Yield quantities, which are given in cup measurements, are accompanied by an approximate number of treatments the recipe will provide.

How much you actually use, of course, will vary. If your hair is long and thick you will use more shampoo than someone with short, thin hair. If you work with

your hands or constantly expose them to the elements, you may find yourself using a lot of hand lotion. Recommendations for usage amounts are, therefore, always approximate.

Storage & Handling

Since PURE BEAUTY preparations contain only natural preservatives, store them carefully to avoid spoilage. Label each with the date it was made and the expiration date (the shelf life is given in each recipe). Discard preparations as they become outdated.

If a recipe doesn't include storage instructions, it is because that recipe is based on active elements of fresh ingredients which will lose potency quickly and must be used immediately.

Resist the temptation to dip your fingers into oil-based creams and lotions, which can contaminate them and cause spoilage. Instead, scoop them out with a cosmetic spatula or tiny spoon.

Many of the ingredients and the products you'll be making must be stored in the refrigerator. This applies particularly to oils and oil-based preparations. which can turn rancid. and to rose water that you plan to store long-term. In general. cool temperatures help to preserve the freshness of creams.

Containers

Some ingredients and preparations. especially products containing essential oils that are going to be kept for more than three months. deteriorate when exposed to light and should be stored in

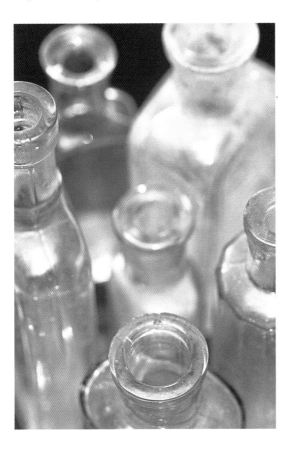

cobalt blue or amber glass containers. Store such potions in a cool, dark place or in the refrigerator. and keep essential oils in small glass vials with tightly fitting caps so they don't evaporate. (See Resources. pages 140-141. for mail-order suppliers of containers.)

A prepared container is clean and dry and has a tight-fitting lid. Before beginning a recipe. make sure you have an appropriately sized bottle or jar set out and ready for filling.

Any container. even a new one. should be washed with a warm deter-gent solution and dried thoroughly with a lint-free cloth before use. One of the pleasures of making your own beauty treatments is displaying them in favorite containers. such as antique glass bottles. If you have jars or bottles you want to reuse—a peanut butter jar for a scrub. an old salt shaker or spice canister with holes in the top for bath salts—wash them thoroughly. then soak them in scalding water for 25 minutes.

Glass storage containers may make beautiful gifts and display pieces, but they are a hazard around the tub and shower. so transfer bathing products to plastic containers before using them.

Precautions

Some of the ingredients called for in this book may cause a slight allergic reaction or minor skin irritation in a very small number of people. Citrus-based preparations, for example, can create photosensitivity or increased sunburn potential in some people, especially those taking certain oral medications.

If you are under medication, regardless of whether it is botanically or synthetically based, consult your physician before using any of the preparations in this book; the herbs may react with the medicine or inhibit its effectiveness.

If you are pregnant, avoid products containing basil, clary sage, clove, juniper berry, marjoram, myrrh, peppermint, rose, rosemary, sage, or thyme essential oils.

In general, you should use the items listed on the opposite page with caution. Test them first, using the skin patch test method described, to see if you react negatively. Negative reactions are extremely rare, but it is important to protect yourself. And always heed the warnings listed with the ingredients in the Glossary (pages 132-139).

If you have very sensitive skin, decrease the amount of essential oils called for by half in any recipe, and be sure to perform a skin patch test.

If you get any solution, preparation, or essential oil in your eyes, immediately wash your eyes by repeatedly flooding them with water. If the irritation continues after washing, consult your physician.

Although many of the ingredients in the recipes are edible, the products themselves are meant for external use only and not for consumption or internal use.

Clearly label all preparations and essential oils and keep them out of the reach of children and pets.

Skin Patch Test

To test for adverse reactions to a substance, make a paste with a half teaspoon of the ingredient and an equal amount of boiling water. Cool the paste to skin temperature, then apply to an area of clean skin on the inside of your forearm near the elbow.

Cover the area with a bandage for 24 hours. If no reaction occurs, proceed with the recipe.

To test essential oils, dilute two drops in one teaspoon of water, saturate a cottonball or pad, and swab on your forearm near the elbow.

If a rash, redness, burning, itching, or irritation occurs, do not use the herb or oil. Consult an herbal expert or aromatherapist about possible substitutions.

If you have sensitive skin or allergies, use the skin patch test before proceeding with any recipes calling for the following ingredients:

Aloe vera
Basil essential oil
Beeswax
Borax
Chamomile
Clove essential oil
Cocoa butter
Fir needle essential oil
Glycerin
Lemon essential oil

Lemongrass essential oil
Orange essential oil
Palm stearic acid
Peppermint essential oil
Spearmint essential oil
Tangerine essential oil
Tea tree essential oil
Vinegar
Vitamin E

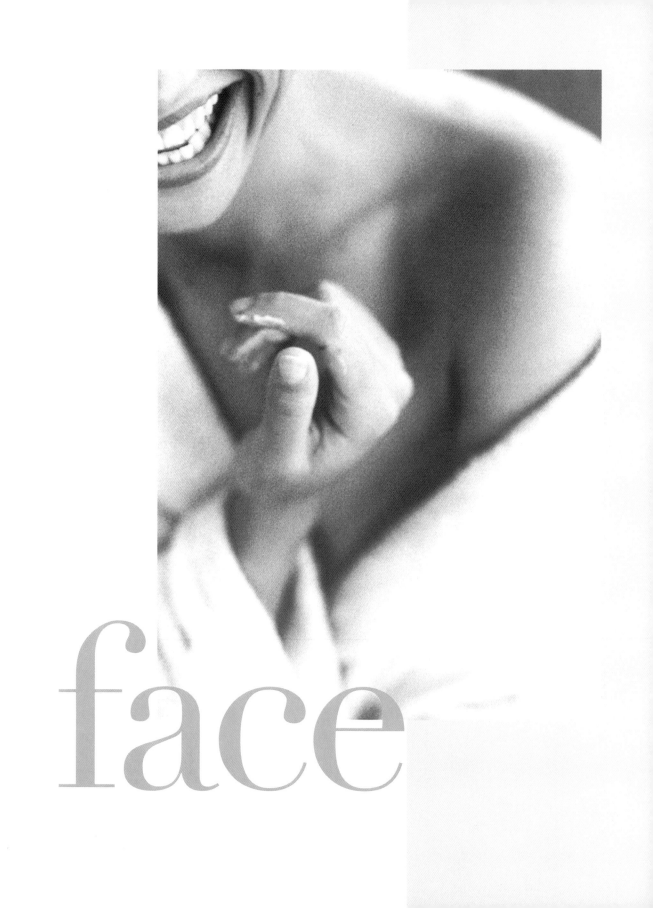

face

Beautiful complexions require care and constant attention: to our exposure to the sun, to what we eat and drink, to the weather, and to the exercise we get. A balanced diet, a proper fitness regimen, and plenty of sunscreen will help keep the face smooth and delay the inevitable signs of aging.

Daily treatments will help, too. Our facial care recipes don't promise to make you immune to wrinkles or blemishes, but they will help keep your face looking and feeling its best.

With nutritious ingredients such as yogurt, almonds, avocado, and apple, the homemade beauty products in this chapter will gently care for the most precious and exposed skin on your body and protect it from the ravages of the environment.

On the following pages you'll find recipes for every stage of a good daily facial care program: cleansers to remove grime and makeup, toners to tighten the look of pores and help eliminate blemishes, moisturizers to rehydrate skin, lip treatments to combat the dryness that comes with wind and sun, and even tooth powders and mouthwashes for healthy teeth and sweet, fresh breath.

For periodic use, or when your skin is troubled, we provide scrubs and exfoliants that gently slough off dead skin cells and make your face glow, masks and face packs to improve your skin's texture, and clarifying lotions for irritated, rashy skin.

Choose facial recipes according to the condition of your skin, taking into consideration your environment and the season. If your skin is normally dry, use a daily cleanser that also moisturizes, such as the Basic Cleansing Milk; if winter weather has your face looking dull or gray, consider a treatment with nourishing properties to stimulate circulation and improve elasticity, like the Creamy Avocado Facial.

When applying exfoliating masks or using cleansing creams, avoid the fragile skin around your eyes. As you cleanse, scrub, or moisturize, be sure to massage gently with an outward, circular motion, and pay attention to the oilier, T-zone formed by your forehead, nose, and chin.

Whatever your skin type, you'll find recipes that will make you feel like the fairest of them all.

face

Basic Cleansing Milk

For centuries, women who have wanted to improve their complexions have used cleansing milk rather than soap. Soap does clean, but it tends to strip the skin of natural oils, leaving it dry and flaky. Cleansing milks, by contrast, are balanced emulsions of oil and water that remove surface grease and dirt, as well as salt left on the skin by perspiration, without upsetting the face's delicate hydro-lipid (water-oil) balance. This cleansing milk is suitable for all skin types.

1. In a mini–food processor or blender, combine the jojoba and avocado oil and blend for 5 seconds. Add the lecithin and blend again for 15 seconds. Add the remaining ingredients and blend for 30 seconds.

2. Transfer the cleansing milk a prepared container and seal tightly. Stored in a refrigerator, it will keep for 3 days. Shake well before using.

2 teaspoons **jojoba**

1 teaspoon **avocado** oil

¼ teaspoon liquid **lecithin**

3 tablespoons whole **milk**

2 tablespoons peeled, seeded, minced **tomato**

2 teaspoons heavy **cream**

1 teaspoon **rosemary** vinegar

3 drops **sweet orange** essential oil

3 drops **ylang-ylang** essential oil

yield

This recipe makes approximately ¼ cup cleansing milk, enough for 2 or 3 cleansings.

to use

Massage onto wet or dry skin with an outward, circular motion, avoiding the sensitive area around the eyes. Rinse with plenty of warm water and pat dry.

Quick Apple & Yogurt Cleanser

In addition to being astringent, apples are full of malic acid and vitamin C, both of which dissolve facial grease and dirt in this easy-to-make cleanser. The enzymes from the active cultures in yogurt are beneficial, too, as they naturally help restore the skin's proper pH balance.

$\frac{1}{8}$ medium-size apple, peeled and cored

2 tablespoons plain yogurt

$\frac{1}{2}$ teaspoon honey

$\frac{1}{2}$ teaspoon lemon juice

$\frac{1}{2}$ teaspoon extra-virgin olive oil

❶ In a blender or mini-food processor, blend the ingredients for about 30 seconds.

❷ Transfer the cleanser to a prepared container and seal tightly. Stored in a refrigerator, it will keep for 4 days.

yield

This recipe makes approximately ¼ cup cleanser, enough for 3 or 4 cleansings.

to use

Scoop out about a tablespoon of cleanser and massage onto dry skin with an outward, circular motion, avoiding the sensitive area around the eyes. Rinse with plenty of warm water and pat dry.

Sweet Orange Cold Cream

The mention of "cold cream" may bring to mind the image of a 1950s housewife slathered in the stuff, but in truth the cool, creamy cleanser has never fallen out of favor. The reason for its enduring popularity is that a cold cream removes grease and dirt but doesn't need to be rinsed off. This version includes sweet orange essential oil—a detoxifier—for a thorough cleansing with a citrusy lift. Enhanced with vitamin E and rose water, it is especially well-suited for combination skin as it will cleanse without drying.

1 In the top of a double boiler, over low heat, melt the beeswax into the olive oil and blend well. Stirring continuously, drizzle in the rose water, then remove from the heat. Continue to stir as the mixture cools. When it has become thick and creamy, stir in the vitamin E and sweet orange essential oil.

2 When the mixture has cooled to room temperature, transfer it to a prepared container and seal tightly. Stored in a cool, dark place, this cold cream will keep for 3 months.

3 tablespoons grated **beeswax**

$\frac{1}{4}$ cup extra-virgin **olive** oil

$\frac{1}{4}$ cup **rose** water

$\frac{1}{2}$ teaspoon **vitamin E**

24 drops **sweet orange** essential oil

yield
This recipe makes approximately ½ cup cold cream, enough for 7 or 8 cleansings.

to use
Scoop out about a tablespoon of cold cream and massage onto dry skin with an outward, circular motion, avoiding the sensitive area around the eyes, and paying particular attention to the "T-zone" (forehead, nose, and chin). Wipe off with a tissue.

Almond & Cornmeal Scrub
for oily skin

Cornmeal's hearty texture and ground almond's gentle sloughing action work together in this recipe to unclog pores, remove dead skin cells, and absorb excess oil released by the action of the scrub. The sumptuous blend of essential oils included here soothes the skin, leaving your face looking and feeling refreshed and healthy.

$^1/_4$ cup finely ground **almonds**

$^1/_4$ cup finely ground white **cornmeal**

1 tablespoon **rose** water

10 drops **lavender** essential oil

5 drops **bergamot** essential oil

3 drops **clary sage** essential oil

1. In a bowl, combine the almonds and cornmeal and blend well. Add the rose water and essential oils, and stir the mixture into a paste.

2. Use immediately.

yield

This recipe makes enough scrub for 1 treatment.

to use

Spread thickly onto wet or dry skin and massage gently with an outward, circular motion, avoiding the sensitive area around the eyes. Leave on for 10 minutes, then rinse off with plenty of warm water. Finish by splashing your face with cold water (to tighten the pores) and pat dry.

Chamomile & Sage Scrub
for sensitive skin

Gently massaging your face with this subtle blend of cleansers and astringents—

oats, almonds, sage, and vinegar—will improve circulation and help the skin release

toxins that could cause blemishes later. Sage is a mild astringent and chamomile

calms the skin, so this scrub is kind enough for even the most sensitive complexions.

1. In a small bowl, combine the ingredients and mix together with your fingers. The mixture will have a dry, grainy consistency.

2. Transfer the scrub to a prepared container and seal tightly. Stored in a refrigerator, it will keep for 3 months.

3 tablespoons ground rolled **oats**

1 tablespoon ground **almonds**

1 tablespoon powdered **chamomile**

1 tablespoon finely ground **sage**

1 tablespoon **apple cider** vinegar

6 drops **chamomile** essential oil

6 drops **sage** essential oil

yield
This recipe makes approximately ½ cup scrub, enough for 6 or 7 treatments.

to use
Spread thickly onto wet or dry skin and massage gently with an outward, circular motion, avoiding the sensitive area around the eyes. Rinse off with plenty of warm water and pat dry.

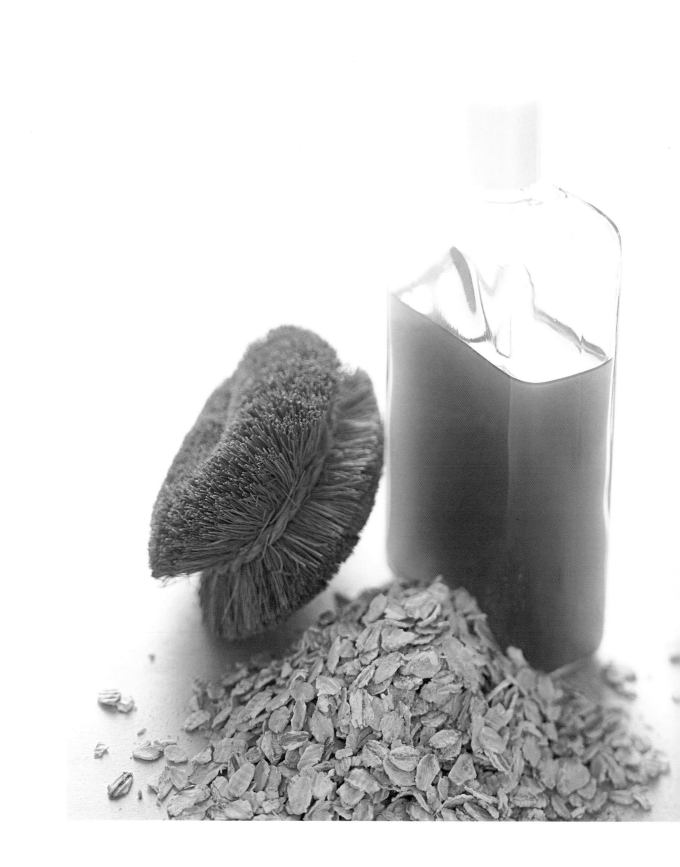

Oats & Honey Mask

Nothing could be simpler than this wonderful toning mask. By gently unblocking pores and improving skin texture, the classic duo of oats and honey restores a natural, healthy glow. If possible, use raw honey and, for best results, make and use this mask as soon as the oatmeal has cooled to room temperature.

1 Combine the oatmeal with the honey and blend to a sticky paste.

2 Use immediately.

$\frac{1}{2}$ cup plain **oatmeal**, cooked and cooled

$\frac{1}{4}$ cup **honey**

yield

This recipe makes enough mask for 1 treatment.

to use

Spread thickly onto skin, avoiding the sensitive area around the eyes. Leave on for 20 minutes, then rinse off with plenty of warm water and pat dry.

Daily Toning Lotion
for oily skin

Anyone prone to oily skin can use this balancing tonic every day. The combination of lavender and calendula with witch hazel will clean and tone while clearing away troublesome blemishes. The essential oils will soothe, soften, and tighten pores.

$1\frac{1}{2}$ cups distilled **water**

$\frac{1}{4}$ cup **calendula** flowers

$\frac{1}{4}$ cup **lavender** flowers and leaves

1 cup **witch hazel** leaves

$\frac{1}{2}$ cup pure **grain alcohol**

4 drops **lavender** essential oil

4 drops **sandalwood** essential oil

2 drops **tea tree** essential oil

yield

This recipe makes approximately 2 cups toning lotion.

to use

Apply lotion to clean, dry skin with a cotton ball or pad.

❶ In a saucepan, over medium heat, combine the water, calendula, and lavender, and bring to a boil. Remove from the heat, cover, and allow to cool for about 1 hour. Strain off and discard the flowers and leaves. Add the witch hazel and alcohol to the infusion.

❷ Pour the mixture into a jar and cap tightly. Refrigerate and shake daily for 2 weeks. Strain the mixture again and add the essential oils.

❸ Transfer the lotion to a prepared container and seal tightly. Stored in a cool, dark place, it will keep for 6 months.

Rose Water Moisturizer

Heady with the fragrance of roses, this silky moisturizer lightly caresses the skin. Although we're recommending it for the face and neck, you could actually use it as a whole-body treatment. So make lots and be lavish; your skin will drink this up.

① In a saucepan, over low heat, combine the rose water, witch hazel, and glycerin. Dissolve the borax into the mixture. When well blended, remove from the heat, cover, and set aside.

② In the top of a double boiler, over low heat, combine the wheat germ oil and jojoba. Melt the beeswax into the mixture and blend well. Slowly whisk in the borax and rose water solution. Continue to whisk as the mixture becomes opaque and begins to thicken, then remove from the heat. Continue whisking as the mixture cools to room temperature, then add the rose otto.

③ Transfer the moisturizer to a prepared container and seal tightly. Stored in a cool, dark place, it will keep for 3 months.

½ cup **rose** water

2 tablespoons **witch hazel** extract

1 tablespoon **glycerin**

¼ teaspoon **borax** powder

2 tablespoons **wheat germ** oil

1 tablespoon **jojoba**

6 tablespoons grated **beeswax**

12 drops **rose otto**

yield

This recipe makes approximately 1 cup moisturizer.

to use

After cleansing and toning, or whenever your skin feels dry, massage a small amount of moisturizer into your face and neck.

Amber Essence Cream

Amber, the golden-brown, translucent resin from the Indian amber tree, has an entrancing fragrance—delicately pungent, enticingly sweet, but not overly sugary. It's a scent that encourages you to slow the pace of life, one that can fill your head with romantic notions. Infused in this rich cream, amber transforms a moisturizer into a perfume. Dab it on sparingly, in strategic places, and breathe deeply.

¼ cup **castor** oil

¼ cup grated **beeswax**

1 tablespoon mashed **amber** resin

¼ cup **rose** water

1 teaspoon **vitamin E**

yield

This recipe makes approximately ¾ cup cream.

to use

After cleansing and toning, or whenever your skin feels dry, massage a small amount of cream into your face and neck.

① In the top of a double boiler, over low heat, add the castor oil and melt the beeswax into it. When well blended, remove the mixture from the heat. Mash the amber with your fingers or in a mortar and pestle and stir it into the melted beeswax and oil. Add the rose water and whisk briskly until the mixture is creamy and forms stiff peaks. Fold in the vitamin E.

② Transfer to a prepared container and seal tightly. Stored in a cool, dark place, this cream will keep for 6 months.

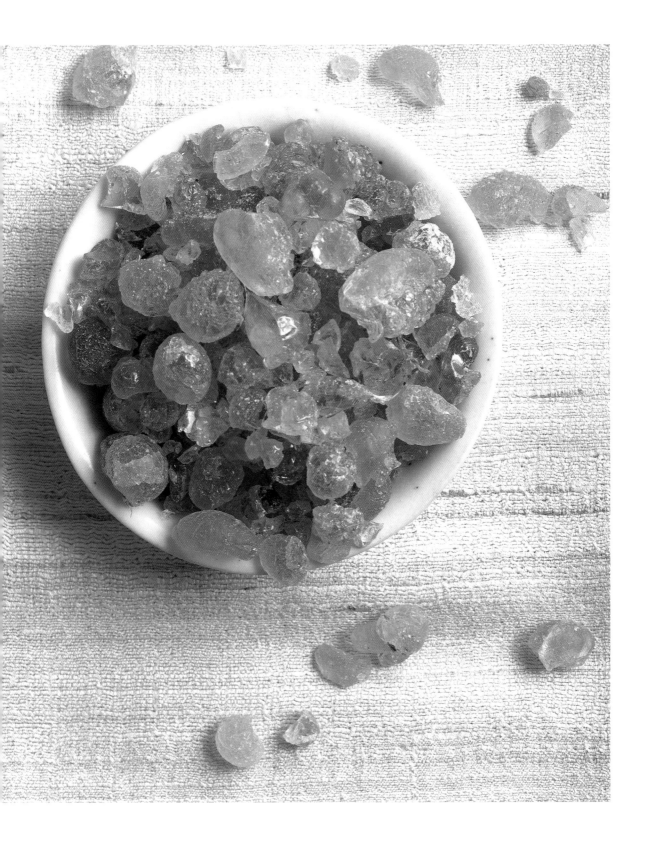

Sweet Almond Eye Cream

Dust and pollution, bright lights and computer screens—it's little wonder our eyes get sore and puffy. For fast relief, splash them with clean, cold water, or recline for ten minutes with cucumber slices on your lids. For a longer-term solution, try this eye cream. With sweet almond oil as a base, it is light and smooth and subtly fragrant. Essential oils soothe and relax overworked muscles around the eyes, and rose water hydrates the thin skin that tends to wrinkle and bag.

¼ cup sweet almond oil

2 tablespoons grated beeswax

3 tablespoons rose water

6 drops vitamin E

4 drops rose otto

4 drops sandalwood essential oil

2 drops lavender essential oil

yield
This recipe makes approximately ½ cup cream.

to use
After cleansing and toning, dab a small amount of cream onto the skin around the eyes.

❶ In the top of a double boiler, over low heat, add the sweet almond oil. Melt the beeswax into the oil and blend well. Stirring continuously, drizzle in the rose water, then remove from the heat. Continue to stir vigorously as the mixture cools and turns thick and creamy. Stir in the vitamin E, rose otto, and the essential oils.

❷ Transfer the cream to a prepared container and seal tightly. Stored in a cool, dark place, it will keep for 3 months.

Sage & Mint Tooth Powder

A sparkling smile might be the most appealing benefit of this recipe, but it's just one of many. Sea salt, baking soda, orange peel, and clay function as mild abrasives, scouring away plaque and leaving teeth clean and bright. Essential oils work to heal sensitive gums; and antibacterial mint essential oils and sage combat bad breath.

1. In a blender or mini–food processor, combine the ingredients and blend until well mixed, about 30 seconds.

2. Transfer the powder to a prepared container and seal tightly. Stored in a cool, dark place, it will keep for 5 days.

2 tablespoons chopped **sage** leaves

1 tablespoon **baking soda**

1 tablespoon finely ground **orange** peel

1 tablespoon powdered **spearmint**

1 tablespoon **white clay**

1 teaspoon fine **sea salt**

2 drops **peppermint** essential oil

1 drop **spearmint** essential oil

yield

This recipe makes approximately ¼ cup tooth powder, enough for 10 to 12 brushings.

to use

Put ½ teaspoon of powder on wax paper. Dip a moistened toothbrush in the powder to coat the bristles, then brush and rinse as you would normally. Do not swallow the powder.

Tea Tree Tooth Powder

If you suffer from bad breath this tooth powder could be your savior. Tea tree essential oil has been used as an antiseptic healing agent for centuries by Australian Aborigines. In this recipe, it reduces tartar, brings the threat of cavities under control, and keeps the bacteria that cause bad breath at bay.

2 tablespoons **green clay**

1 tablespoon **baking soda**

1 tablespoon fine **sea salt**

4 drops **tea tree** essential oil

2 drops **spearmint** essential oil

1. In a blender or mini-food processor, combine the ingredients and blend until well mixed, about 30 seconds.

2. Transfer the powder to a prepared container and seal tightly. Stored in a cool, dark place, it will keep for 4 days.

yield

This recipe makes approximately ¼ cup tooth powder, enough for 10 to 12 brushings.

to use

Put ½ teaspoon of powder on wax paper. Dip a moistened toothbrush in the powder to coat the bristles, then brush and rinse as you would normally. Do not swallow the powder.

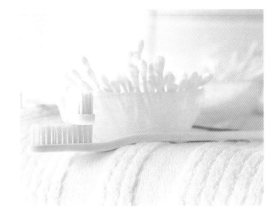

Sage & Witch Hazel Mouthwash

Chewing on a sprig of mint or parsley after a meal will freshen your breath. but this mouthwash has the added medicinal benefits of sage. which has long been used for treating gingivitis and restoring good gum health. and witch hazel. which soothes and heals canker sores. Use witch hazel extract made with grain alcohol: other varieties may contain harmful chemicals.

1. In a food processor or blender. combine the ingredients and blend for 1 minute. Strain and discard the solids.

2. Transfer the mouthwash to a prepared bottle and cap tightly. Stored in a cool. dark place. it will keep for up to 5 days.

$^3/_4$ cup distilled **water**

$^1/_4$ cup **witch hazel** extract

3 tablespoons **mint**

3 tablespoons **parsley**

3 tablespoons **sage**

1 tablespoon pure **grain alcohol**

yield

This recipe makes approximately
1 cup mouthwash, enough for
6 or 7 rinses.

to use

After brushing, swirl a few teaspoons
of mouthwash around your mouth
for 30 seconds or so, then spit out.
Do not swallow the mouthwash.

Cinnamon & Clove Mouthwash

Aromatic spices combine with fragrant sweet orange essential oil to create a mild, cleansing mouthwash that will give your breath long-lasting freshness. For good measure, tea tree essential oil provides an antibacterial boost.

$^1\!/_4$ teaspoon ground cinnamon

$^1\!/_4$ teaspoon ground cloves

$^1\!/_4$ teaspoon ground fennel seeds

$^1\!/_4$ teaspoon ground star anise

$^1\!/_2$ cup pure grain alcohol

$1^1\!/_2$ cups distilled water

20 drops sweet orange essential oil

6 drops tea tree essential oil

1 In a jar, combine the spices and alcohol. Seal tightly and refrigerate for 3 days. Strain off and discard the solids. Add the water and essential oils.

2 Transfer the mouthwash to a prepared container and seal tightly. Stored in a cool, dark place, it will keep for 3 months.

yield

This recipe makes approximately 2 cups mouthwash, enough for 12 to 14 rinses.

to use

After brushing, swirl a few teaspoons of mouthwash around your mouth for 30 seconds or so, then spit out. Do not swallow the mouthwash.

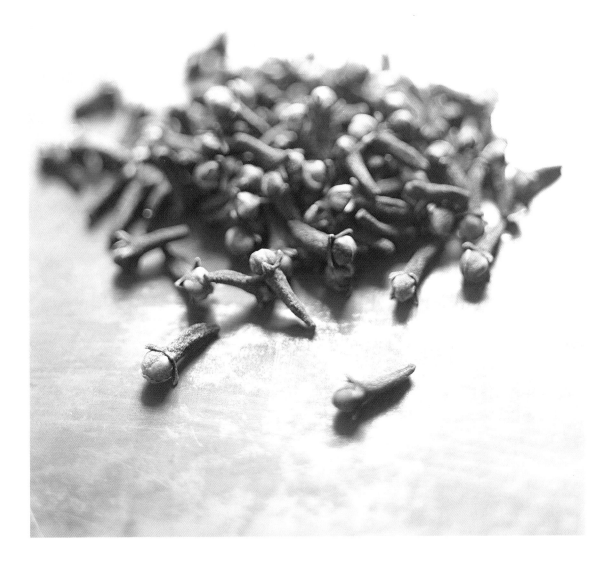

Unscented Lip Gloss

Protective, moisturizing, and conditioning, this lip gloss will make your lips soft and shiny without adding scent or color. The blend becomes semisolid, rather like an ointment; if you prefer a firmer version, add an extra half-teaspoon grated beeswax.

3 tablespoons castor oil

1 tablespoon jojoba

2 tablespoons grated beeswax

1 teaspoon honey

¼ teaspoon vitamin E

① In the top of a double boiler, over low heat, combine the castor oil and jojoba. Stir the beeswax into the mixture. When well blended, remove from the heat, and stir in the honey and vitamin E.

② Transfer the gloss to a prepared container and seal tightly. Stored in a cool, dark place, it will keep for 3 months.

yield

This recipe makes approximately ¼ cup lip gloss.

to use

With a clean finger or lip brush, apply to your lips whenever they feel dry or sore.

Filling Lip-Balm Tubes

1. Fill a small, two-inch-deep baking pan halfway with a layer of uncooked lentils, small beans, or sand.

2. In the lentils, stand the tubes straight up so their bases are flat against the pan bottom and the lentils are holding the tubes firmly in place.

3. Using a turkey baster with a squeeze bulb, draw up the melted lip balm and squirt it gently into each lip balm tube.

4. Let cool until balm becomes solid.

Almond & Jojoba Lip Butter

Both winter wind and summer sun will dry and crack lips, so this healing balm is perfect for anyone who loves to spend time outdoors. Vitamin E and jojoba possess excellent moisturizing qualities, sweet almond oil and beeswax form a protective coating to help prevent moisture loss, and tea tree and lavender essential oils heal chapped lips.

1. In the top of a double boiler, over low heat, combine the glycerin, sweet almond oil, and jojoba. Melt the beeswax into the mixture. When well blended, remove from the heat, and stir in the vitamin E and the essential oils.

2. Transfer the lip butter to a prepared container and seal tightly. Stored in a cool, dark place, it will keep for 3 months.

3 tablespoons **glycerin**

3 tablespoons **sweet almond** oil

1 tablespoon **jojoba**

1/4 cup grated **beeswax**

1/4 teaspoon **vitamin E**

2 drops **lavender** essential oil

2 drops **tea tree** essential oil

yield

This recipe makes about 1/2 cup lip butter.

to use

With a clean finger or lip brush, apply to your lips whenever they feel dry or sore.

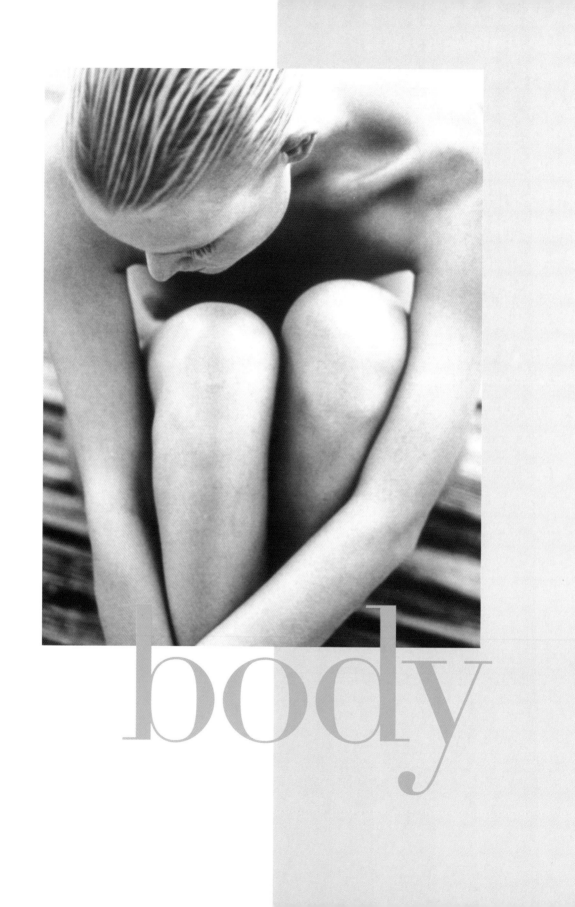

body

Nothing is as enticing as soft, smooth, polished skin. Covering an area of more than eighteen square feet, skin is our largest organ. It protects us in our daily contact with the world and the elements, but we also must protect it.

Drinking lots of clean water helps flush out toxins that otherwise might surface as blemishes. Applying moisturizing lotion helps skin stay supple by maintaining its elasticity, which diminishes with age. Sloughing off dead cells with a scrub or an exfoliating polish clears clogged pores, prevents dead cells from accumulating, and enables new cells to get the nourishment they need to create pure, beautiful, radiant skin.

How you live affects the condition of your skin. Protect yourself from ultraviolet rays on sunny days by using a good sunscreen and staying covered. Wear cotton, silk, and other natural fabrics against your skin (tight synthetics can cause irritations). A healthful diet, fresh air, and stimulating exercise make an enormous difference in how your skin looks and feels.

Many of the recipes in this chapter are for bath and shower products—treatments for skin that also work wonders for your state of mind. You'll find lotions that soften skin and aid circulation; calming, cleansing gels; aromatic bubble baths; herbal bath oils and salts; and body scrubs.

Unlike chemically based preparations, these natural products are scented with herbs, flowers, and essential oils, giving them nourishing and aromatherapeutic properties. Because the recipes use only pure glycerin or castile soap, you'll find the suds in your homemade bubble baths smaller and less bouncy—but far more effective—than those in synthetic formulas.

Baths are the best way for your body to absorb the benefits of natural ingredients such as herbs, salts, and moisturizing oils because skin is most receptive when it's warm and damp. Plus, soaking is soothing—what could be more relaxing than lying in a tub of soft, milky water scented with aromatic lavender? So make time to sit and soak, letting your mind wander. Just avoid very hot water, since extreme temperatures can dry your skin.

A regular body scrub with a good exfoliant stimulates the circulatory system while helping skin shed dead cells. Whether you're using your hands or a loofah to rub, the motion should be made toward the heart, where blood circulation originates.

To augment your beauty regime, slather yourself with one of the rich lotions, creams, or oils in this chapter right after you bathe or shower. For a special treat, finish your bath routine with a dab of a fragrant cream, such as Jasmine Cream Perfume, to keep your body smelling as good as it feels.

Lavender & Rosemary Milk Bath

Washing becomes a decadent and heady experience in this fragrant, creamy bath. As you soak, rich buttermilk powder dissolves into salt-softened water, moisturizing your skin and calming your nerves. Rosemary gently stimulates the circulatory and respiratory systems, helping to release unwanted body toxins. And aromatic lavender soothes away the tensions of the day, leaving you feeling dreamy and peaceful.

½ cup powdered **buttermilk**

½ cup **Epsom salts**

½ cup nonfat powdered **milk**

½ cup fine **sea salt**

¼ cup coarse **kosher salt**

1 teaspoon powdered **lavender**

1 teaspoon powdered **rosemary**

1 In a food processor or blender, combine the ingredients and blend well.

2 Transfer the mixture to a prepared container and seal tightly. Kept dry in a cool, dark place, this milk bath will stay fresh for 1 month.

yield

This recipe makes approximately 2½ cups milk bath, enough for 6 or 7 baths.

to use

Add about ⅓ cup of milk bath to running water as your bath fills.

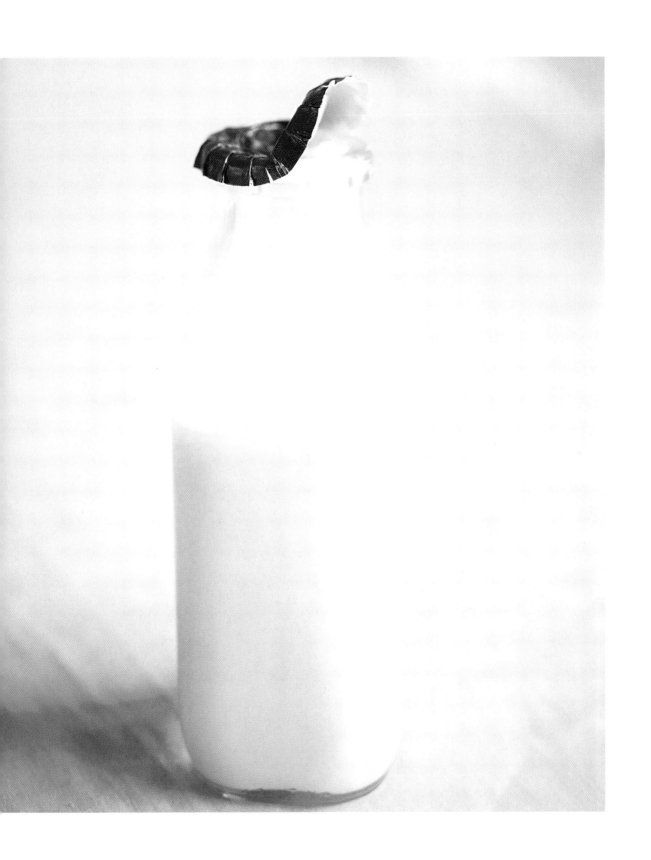

Herb Garden Bath & Shower Gel

¼ cup **rose** water

1 tablespoon dried **chamomile** leaves and flowers

1 tablespoon dried **peppermint**

1 tablespoon dried **rose** petals

1 tablespoon dried **sage** blossoms or leaves

½ cup **glycerin** soap base

1 teaspoon **castor** oil

12 drops **sandalwood** essential oil

6 drops **lavender** essential oil

4 drops **geranium bourbon** essential oil

yield

This recipe makes approximately ½ cup bath gel, enough for 2 or 3 baths.

to use

Squirt the gel under running water as your bath fills, or use it as a cleansing gel with a puff or loofah sponge.

The scent of an herb garden will come wafting up as you smooth this fragrant cleansing gel over your body. Soft and cooling. it contains essential oils that calm. center. and relax, easing you into the morning or relieving stress in the evening.

1 In a saucepan. heat the rose water. Before it boils. remove from the heat and add the chamomile. peppermint. rose petals. and sage blossoms. Cover and let steep for 1 hour.

2 Strain off and discard the solids. Then, over low heat, gently reheat the rose water. Add the glycerin soap and castor oil. Once the glycerin has melted. add the essential oils and blend well.

3 Cover the gel and let cool to room temperature. Transfer it to a prepared container and seal tightly. Stored in a refrigerator. this gel will keep for 7 to 10 days.

Rose Geranium Bubble Bath

Used for centuries in skin-care preparations. geranium soothes and rebalances. so it is especially good for dry. sensitive skin. Rosewood has properties similar to geranium. and they team up here to create a softly foaming bubble bath with an entrancing floral aroma.

1 In a bowl. combine the castile soap and the rose water. When well blended. add the glycerin. salt. and the essential oils. Stir until well mixed.

2 Transfer the bubble bath to a prepared container and seal tightly. Stored in a cool. dark place. it will keep for 1 year.

2 cups liquid castile soap

1/2 cup rose water

2 tablespoons glycerin

1 teaspoon sea salt

30 drops rose geranium essential oil

8 drops rosewood essential oil

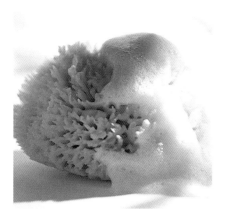

yield

This recipe makes approximately 1 cup bath gel, enough for 5 or 6 baths.

to use

Squirt the bubble bath under running water as your bath fills, or use it as a cleansing gel with a puff or loofah sponge.

Herbal Bath Sachets

Herbal sachets are a sensational way to add the many benefits of herbs to a bath: Just fill little muslin drawstring bags, available at craft shops and herb stores, with your favorite herbs and hang them under the faucet as the bath fills. The herbal aroma and nutrients will filter into the water, then be absorbed into your skin. You can also exfoliate with the sachets themselves; brushing one over your skin lifts away dead cells and stimulates the release of toxins. We've suggested some blends on the opposite page. It's not necessary to use all the herbs in a blend, you can mix and match what you have available and borrow from other blends if you like.

Use chopped fresh herbs or gently crumbled dried herbs for the bath bags. Avoid powdered herbs as they can clog the muslin and inhibit the other herbs from steeping properly. For additional skin-softening properties, add one-quarter cup of any the following ingredients to your herbal mix: oatmeal, cornmeal, coarsely ground almonds, bath salts, or powdered milk.

2 tablespoons each of at least 4 selected **herbs**

yield
Regular sachets will hold about ½ cup herbs.

to use
Hang the bag over the bathtub top so that the water runs through it, or toss the bag directly into the tub and swirl it around.

① In a bowl, combine the ingredients and blend well.

② Spoon the mixture into prepared muslin bags. Draw and tie off the strings.

③ Stored in an airtight container, these bath sachets will stay fresh for 6 months.

For oily skin

comfrey root, eucalyptus, geranium leaves, lavender flowers, lemongrass, nettles, orange leaves, patchouli leaves, peppermint, raspberry leaves, rosemary, sage, spearmint, thyme, white willow bark, witch hazel bark and leaves, yarrow flowers

For dry skin

calendula petals, chamomile flowers, fennel seeds, honeysuckle flowers, orange flowers, rose petals, ylang-ylang flowers

To exfoliate

comfrey root, nettle leaves, sage, white oak bark, witch hazel leaves, yarrow flowers

To soften

calendula petals, honeysuckle flowers, linden flowers, Queen Anne's lace flowers, rose petals

To tone

lavender flowers, mint, patchouli leaves, thyme, yarrow flowers

Nourishing Bath Oil

Feed your skin this nourishing oil. Because it floats on the surface of the bathwater, it will coat your body as you enter and leave the tub, but it will not leave you feeling oily or greasy. The highly aromatic essential oils blend musky earth scents with sweet florals: they come from herbs that stimulate the sebaceous glands, which properly regulate the skin's moisture level.

2 tablespoons avocado oil

2 tablespoons castor oil

2 tablespoons sweet almond oil

2 tablespoons wheat germ oil

8 drops ylang-ylang essential oil

6 drops sandalwood essential oil

4 drops fir needle essential oil

3 drops patchouli essential oil

2 drops lavender essential oil

1 In a prepared container, combine the ingredients, seal tightly, and shake gently to blend.

2 Stored in a refrigerator, this bath oil will keep for 3 months. Shake before using.

yield

This recipe makes approximately ½ cup bath oil, enough for 24 to 26 baths.

to use

Add about 1 teaspoon of bath oil to your bathwater before sliding in to soak. After getting out of the bath, but before toweling dry, rub the oil into your skin, especially into areas that are prone to dryness.

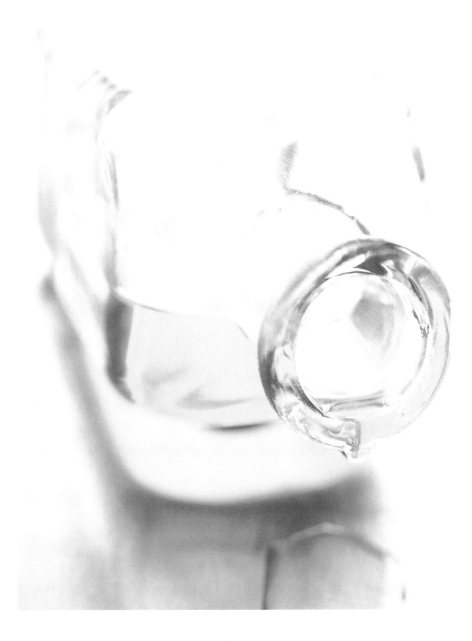

Disappearing Bath Oil

This bath oil disappears into the water — instead of floating on the surface — to be readily absorbed by the skin. Sweet almond oil is light and almost odorless and, combined with glycerin and castile soap, easily disperses through water. To this combination, add your favorite essential oils, or choose one of the suggested blends on the opposite page. Then slip into an essential oil-infused bath and feel your tensions disappear, too.

1 cup **sweet almond** oil

$\frac{1}{2}$ cup **glycerin**

$\frac{1}{2}$ cup liquid **castile soap**

1 **essential oil** blend

yield

This recipe makes approximately 2 cups bath oil, enough for 7 or 8 baths.

to use

Pour ¼ cup of bath oil under running water as your bath fills.

1. In a bowl, combine the ingredients and blend well.

2. Transfer the bath oil to a prepared container and seal tightly. Stored in a refrigerator, it will keep for 6 months. Shake before using.

Relaxing
Essential Oil Blends

36 drops chamomile essential oil
24 drops cedarwood essential oil
24 drops fennel essential oil
16 drops cypress essential oil

32 drops spruce essential oil
24 drops lavender essential oil
20 drops cypress essential oil
20 drops dill essential oil

28 drops sandalwood essential oil
20 drops chamomile essential oil
16 drops cedarwood essential oil
12 drops cajeput essential oil
12 drops cypress essential oil

16 drops sandalwood essential oil
10 drops lemon essential oil
10 drops spruce essential oil
6 drops dill essential oil
6 drops fennel essential oil

10 drops chamomile essential oil
10 drops lavender essential oil
10 drops lemongrass essential oil
8 drops cypress essential oil

Stimulating
Essential Oil Blends

32 drops geranium bourbon essential oil
24 drops rosemary essential oil
16 drops peppermint essential oil
8 drops ginger essential oil

32 drops bergamot essential oil
24 drops rosemary essential oil
16 drops lime essential oil
16 drops patchouli essential oil
16 drops spearmint essential oil

24 drops bergamot essential oil
24 drops rosewood essential oil
24 drops lime essential oil
16 drops ylang-ylang essential oil
12 drops eucalyptus essential oil

14 drops lime essential oil
12 drops spearmint essential oil
10 drops juniper essential oil
6 drops eucalyptus essential oil
6 drops ginger essential oil

12 drops bergamot essential oil
12 drops grapefruit essential oil
10 drops ylang-ylang essential oil
8 drops patchouli essential oil
6 drops peppermint essential oil

Basic Bath Salts

Long ago, people noticed that the water below and around salt deposits seemed softer and more healing to the body. Thus began the now-ancient tradition of adding salt to the waters in bathhouses, along with fragrant herbal and floral distillations for elegant aromas. Bath salts may seem old-fashioned, but they are still the quickest and most effective way to neutralize the trace elements that harden tap water and, by extension, your skin. See which of the blends on the opposite page works best with your skin condition, then make up a batch of salts to keep by the tub.

1 cup coarse or fine **sea salt**

1 cup **Epsom salts**

¼ cup **glycerin**

1 **essential oil** blend

yield
This recipe makes approximately 2 cups bath salts, enough for 4 baths.

to use
Add ½ cup of bath salts to running water as your bath fills and swirl to dissolve.

❶ In a bowl, combine the salts and the glycerin. When well blended, stir in the essential oil blend. Let stand for 15 minutes.

❷ Transfer the salts to a prepared container and seal tightly. Stored in a sealed container, they will stay fresh for 1 year.

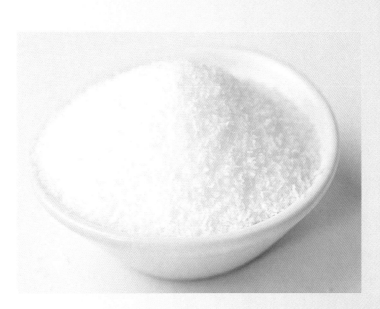

For toning and well-being

20 drops geranium bourbon essential oil

16 drops spearmint essential oil

12 drops oregano essential oil

12 drops thyme essential oil

For sensitive skin

16 drops lavender essential oil

12 drops chamomile essential oil

12 drops fir essential oil

8 drops cypress essential oil

For oily skin

12 drops cypress essential oil

12 drops peppermint essential oil

8 drops eucalyptus essential oil

8 drops sage essential oil

8 drops valerian essential oil

For tired-looking skin

12 drops cajeput essential oil

12 drops lavender essential oil

12 drops lemongrass essential oil

8 drops eucalyptus essential oil

Sweet Citrus Body Polish

Even in the middle of winter, the sweet, tangy aroma of this body scrub will remind you of sunny citrus groves. We call it a polish because the sloughing action of the salts, combined with the moisturizing effect of the jojoba and sweet almond oil, results in silky, gleaming skin.

$\frac{3}{4}$ cup liquid castile soap

$\frac{3}{4}$ cup jojoba

2 tablespoons sweet almond oil

$\frac{1}{2}$ cup fine sea salt

2 tablespoons coarse sea salt

$\frac{1}{2}$ teaspoon sweet orange essential oil

$\frac{1}{2}$ teaspoon tangerine essential oil

10 drops neroli essential oil

1. In a bowl, combine the castile soap, jojoba, and sweet almond oil and blend well. Add the fine and coarse sea salts, and the essential oils. Blend again.

2. Transfer the polish to a prepared container, preferably a wide-mouth jar so you can easily scoop it out. Seal tightly. Stored in a cool, dry place, this body polish will keep for 1 year.

yield

This recipe makes approximately 2 cups body polish, enough for 7 or 8 baths or showers.

to use

Scoop up a handful of polish and slather over your body in the bath or shower.

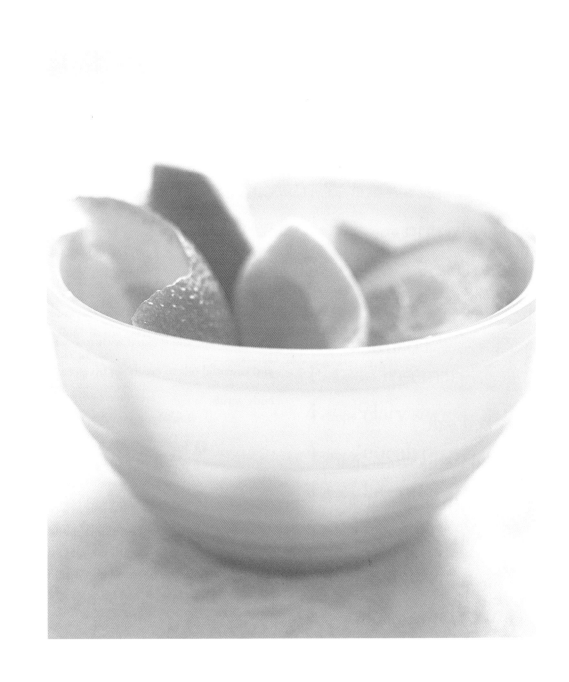

Moisturizing Amber Scrub

Amber is sold in small chunks at good herb and incense supply stores. Just mash it up with your fingers and blend it into this scrub. Then breathe in deeply: its special aroma will transport you as you scrub.

¼ cup glycerin soap base

2 tablespoons sweet almond oil

¼ cup jojoba

¼ cup medium sea salt

2 tablespoons mashed amber resin

yield
Makes approximately ¾ cup scrub, enough for 3 or 4 treatments.

to use
Scoop up a handful of scrub and slather over your body in the bath or shower.

1. In the top of a double boiler, over low heat, melt the glycerin soap with the sweet almond oil and jojoba, and blend well. Then slowly stir in the salt. Remove from the heat and mix in the amber.

2. Transfer the scrub to a prepared container, preferably a wide-mouth jar, and seal tightly. Stored in a cool, dry place, it will keep for 3 months.

Ylang-Ylang Lotion Bar

Here delicate, moisturizing oils blend with beeswax to form a solid bar that looks like soap but feels like a soft candle. The bar is scented with ylang-ylang essential oil, which normalizes the activities of the glands so they don't secrete too much or too little oil.

For bar molds you could use soap molds, the plastic drawer organizers available in supermarkets and discount stores, or small boxes lined with plastic wrap.

1. In the top of a double boiler, over low heat, melt the beeswax and the cocoa butter with the coconut oil, jojoba, wheat germ oil, and the vitamin E, and blend well. Mix in the ylang-ylang and geranium bourbon essential oils.

2. Pour the lotion into a prepared mold and allow to cool and harden.

3. When completely cool, carefully remove the bar from the mold and transfer it to an airtight container. Stored in a refrigerator, a lotion bar will keep for 1 year.

1 cup grated **beeswax**

¼ cup **cocoa butter**

¼ cup **coconut** oil

¼ cup **jojoba**

¼ cup **wheat germ** oil

½ teaspoon **vitamin E**

10 drops **ylang-ylang** essential oil

4 drops **geranium bourbon** essential oil

yield

This recipe makes the equivalent of approximately 1 cup lotion.

to use

Warm the bar in your hands, then rub it over your skin, massaging in as necessary.

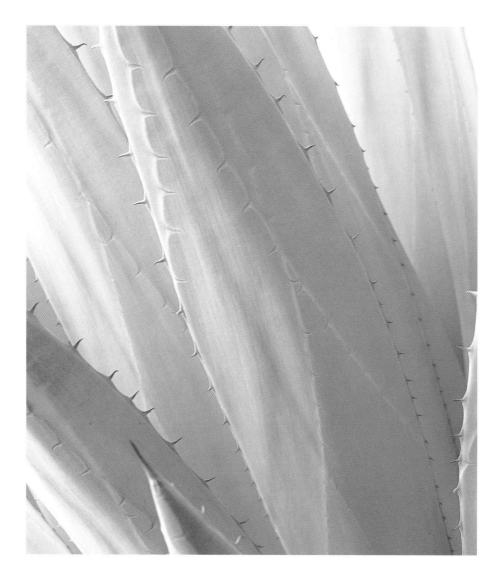

Aloe Vera & Witch Hazel Toning Lotion

Witch hazel has long been believed to diminish varicose and spider veins. In this lotion it is combined with aloe vera, which acts as a detoxifier, and vitamin E, which nourishes healthy cell growth, to stimulate and revitalize the blood flow in your legs.

1. In the top of a double boiler, over low heat, melt the beeswax with the olive oil, shea butter, and palm stearic acid, and blend well. Remove the mixture from the heat and whisk in the vitamin E, aloe vera, witch hazel, and glycerin. Continue whisking until the lotion looks creamy.

2. Transfer the lotion to a prepared container and seal tightly. Stored in a cool, dry place, it will keep for 6 weeks.

2 tablespoons grated beeswax

¼ cup extra-virgin olive oil

¼ cup shea butter

1 tablespoon palm stearic acid

1 tablespoon vitamin E

¼ cup aloe vera gel

¼ cup witch hazel extract

1 teaspoon glycerin

yield

This recipe makes approximately 1 cup toning lotion.

to use

Massage lotion into clean, dry skin after bathing, especially where skin is irritated or veins are visible.

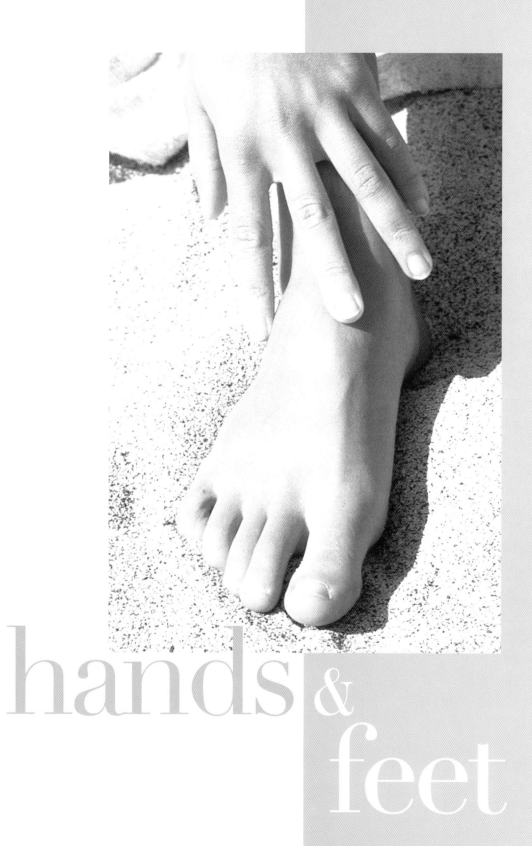

hands & feet

Every day our hands are assailed by the demands of daily living: sun and wind, frigid and scalding water, detergents and household cleaners, and the scrapes, cuts, and pinpricks we suffer in the kitchen, office, or workroom. Our feet, meanwhile, carry the weight of our bodies and are subjected to shoes that rub, pinch, burn, and trap moisture. But despite the abuse our hands and feet take, we tend to neglect them—that is, until we bare our callused feet in the first days of summer, or take a good look at our rough, red hands or brittle, chipped nails before a special occasion. By then, of course, it's too late; there are no quick fixes. Beautiful hands and feet need regular maintenance and care.

Lemon & Tangerine Hand Cream

After doing the dishes or washing the car, combat the harsh effects of detergents with this rich hand cream. Lemon essential oil is antiseptic and helps eliminate germs and odors, while tangerine (or mandarin) essential oil is a superb skin conditioner that smooths and softens hands.

½ teaspoon borax

½ cup rose water

¼ cup grated beeswax

¼ cup avocado oil

¼ cup jojoba

1 tablespoon honey

1 teaspoon vitamin E

30 drops tangerine or mandarin essential oil

20 drops lemon essential oil

yield

This recipe makes approximately 1 cup hand cream.

to use

Massage a generous amount into hands after washing or whenever they feel dry.

❶ In a small bowl, combine the borax and the rose water. Dissolve the borax, and set aside.

❷ In the top of a double boiler, over low heat, melt the beeswax with the avocado oil, jojoba, and honey, and blend well. Stir in the vitamin E.

❸ Transfer the mixture to a blender or mini–food processor. With the blender set on low, drizzle in the rose water–borax mixture. Switch the blender to high until the mixture looks thick and creamy, about 30 seconds. Pour the cream into a clean bowl and whisk in the essential oils until well blended.

❹ Transfer the cream to a prepared container and seal tightly. Stored in a refrigerator, it will keep for 3 months.

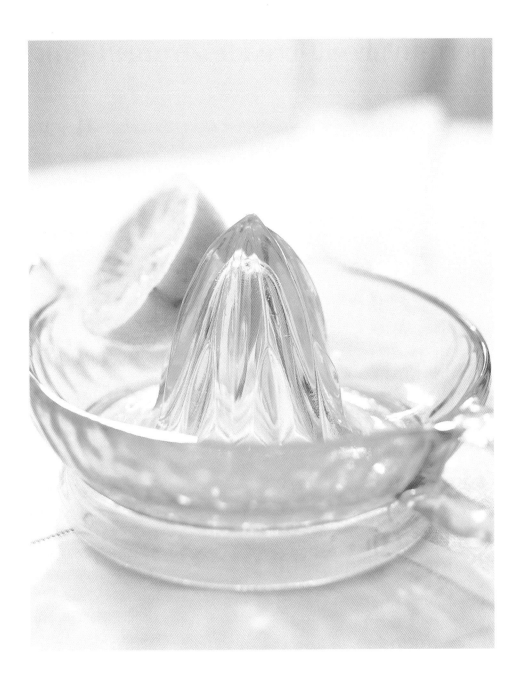

Patchouli & Rose Hand Oil

When your hands are dry and cracked but you don't have time to soak them, this oil could very well be your savior. A few drops provide instant relief, absorbing into the skin immediately without leaving any residue.

¼ cup jojoba

¼ cup vitamin E

12 drops patchouli essential oil

10 drops rose otto

8 drops geranium bourbon
    essential oil

8 drops lemon essential oil

1. Combine the ingredients in a prepared container, seal tightly, and shake well.

2. Stored in a cool, dry place, this oil will keep for 1 year. Shake before using.

yield
This recipe makes approximately ½ cup oil.

to use
Massage a few drops into your hands after washing or whenever they feel dry.

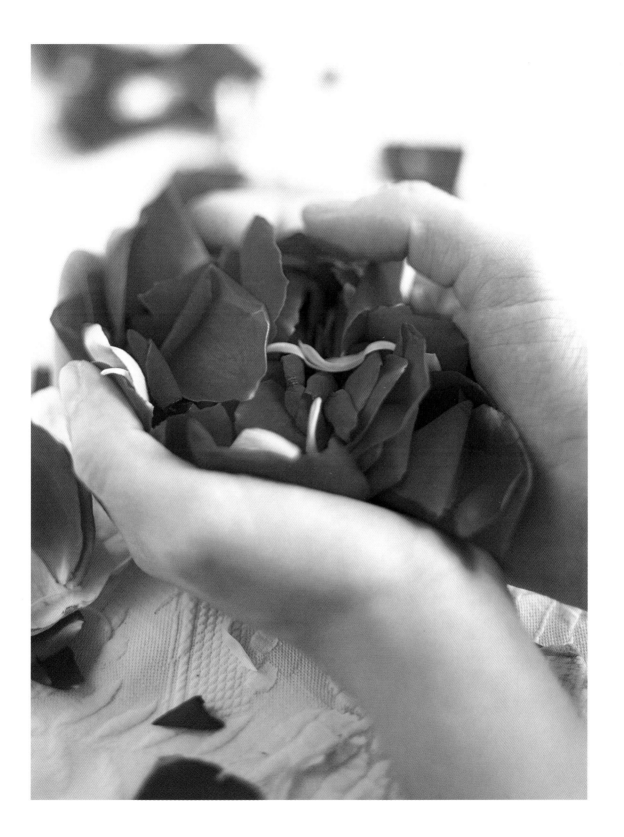

Sandalwood Hand Oil

Sandalwood oil has long been revered for its emollient and anti-inflammatory properties. It is known to alleviate dry, irritated skin, and aromatherapists believe it centers the soul.

¼ cup jojoba

¼ cup wheat germ oil

2 tablespoons evening primrose oil

2 tablespoons extra-virgin olive oil

2 tablespoons vitamin E

18 drops carrot seed essential oil

18 drops sandalwood essential oil

4 drops geranium bourbon essential oil

4 drops lemon essential oil

4 drops patchouli essential oil

① Combine the ingredients in a prepared container, seal tightly, and shake well.

② Stored in a cool, dark place, this oil will keep for 1 year. Shake before using.

yield

This recipe makes approximately 1 cup oil.

to use

Massage a few drops into your hands after washing or whenever they feel dry.

Lemon & Rosewood Rubbing Oil

Here is an easy, effective treatment for dry, troubled hands and feet—particularly those prone to calluses and cramping. This oil is not greasy and will readily penetrate the skin. The action of rubbing and massaging relaxes muscles and stimulates hands and feet to absorb the nourishing oils.

1 Combine the ingredients in a prepared container, seal tightly, and shake well.

2 Stored in a cool, dry place, this rubbing oil will keep for 2 years. Shake before using.

¼ cup jojoba

12 drops lemon essential oil

10 drops rosewood essential oil

8 drops palma rosa essential oil

4 drops thyme essential oil

yield

This recipe makes approximately ¼ cup oil.

to use

Massage directly into callused areas or rub some across the whole hand or foot.

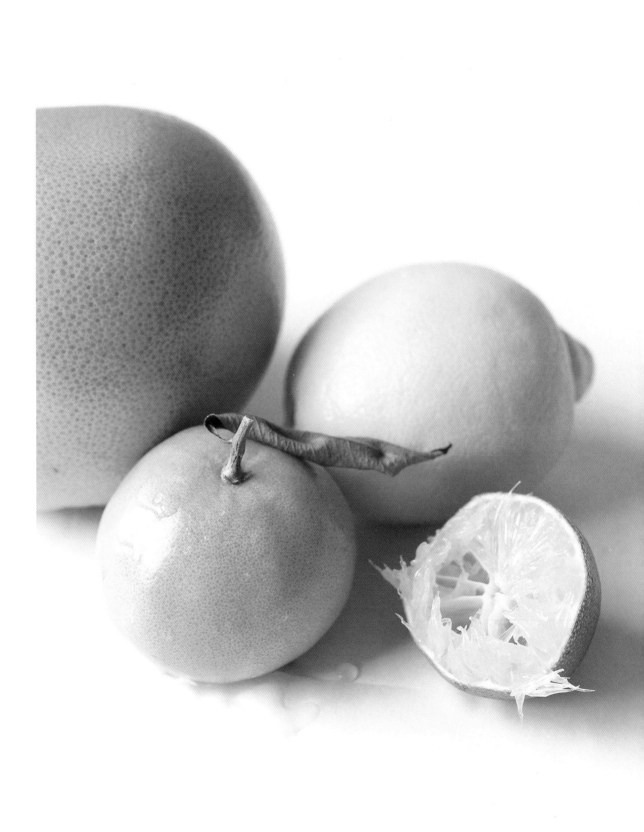

Citrus Balm
for calluses

Calluses that build up on your feet can be difficult to get rid of and even more difficult to live with. This citrus balm softens the hard, dry skin that causes foot discomfort, and provides vital nutrients to the live cells underneath.

1 In the top of a double boiler, over low heat, melt the beeswax with the coconut oil. When blended, remove the mixture from the heat and add the jojoba, wheat germ oil, lecithin, and borax. Whisk in the orange floral water and the essential oils. The mixture will get very thick, but keep mixing until blended.

2 Allow the balm to cool and transfer it to a prepared container, preferably a wide-mouth jar. Seal tightly. Stored in a cool, dark place, this balm will last for 3 months.

2 tablespoons grated **beeswax**

2 tablespoons **coconut** oil

2 tablespoons **jojoba**

2 tablespoons **wheat germ** oil

1 teaspoon **lecithin**

$\frac{1}{8}$ teaspoon **borax**

2 tablespoons **orange** floral water

15 drops **sweet orange** essential oil

5 drops **lime** essential oil

5 drops **tangerine** essential oil

yield
This recipe makes approximately ¾ cup balm.

to use
Massage a generous amount into calluses daily.

Winter Hand Balm

Snow, ice, wind, even tight gloves can all wreak havoc on your hands. To counteract the effects of a winter day's weather, apply a generous amount of this nutrient-rich balm before bed and leave on your hands overnight.

$\frac{1}{2}$ teaspoon **baking soda**

$\frac{3}{4}$ cup **rose** water

$\frac{1}{4}$ cup grated **beeswax**

$\frac{1}{4}$ cup **palm stearic** acid

$\frac{1}{4}$ cup **avocado** oil

$\frac{1}{4}$ cup **jojoba**

$\frac{1}{4}$ cup **wheat germ** oil

1 tablespoon **aloe vera** oil

1 teaspoon **vitamin E**

16 drops **lavender** essential oil

4 drops **geranium bourbon** essential oil

1 In a small bowl, dissolve the baking soda in the rose water, and set aside.

2 In the top of a double boiler, over low heat, melt the beeswax and palm stearic acid with the avocado oil, jojoba, wheat germ oil, and aloe vera oil. Blend well. Drizzle one third of the rose water solution into the beeswax mixture. Mix well. Transfer the mixture to a blender and, with the blender on high, drizzle in the remaining two thirds of the rose water solution. When the mixture begins to thicken, add the vitamin E and the essential oils, and blend for a few more seconds.

3 Transfer the balm to a prepared container and allow to cool completely before sealing tightly. Stored in a cool place, it will keep for 4 months.

yield
This recipe makes approximately 2 cups moisturizing balm.

to use
Massage a generous amount into your hands before bed or whenever they feel cold and dry.

Calendula & Chamomile Foot Balm

Calendula is prized for its moisturizing and muscle-soothing properties, while chamomile is a natural, mild sedative with a relaxing effect on the body's tissues.

1. In a small saucepan, over low heat, simmer the powdered calendula and chamomile flowers and the olive oil for 1 hour. Stir in the beeswax until melted. Add the essential oils and remove the mixture from the heat.

2. Transfer the balm to a prepared container, seal tightly, and allow to cool. Stored in a cool, dark place, it will keep for 4 months.

1 teaspoon powdered **calendula** flowers

1 teaspoon powdered **chamomile** flowers

1/2 cup extra-virgin **olive** oil

3 tablespoons grated **beeswax**

20 drops **tea tree** essential oil

8 drops **lavender** essential oil

4 drops **rosemary** essential oil

4 drops **sage** essential oil

Herbal Nail-Growth Blend

It takes more than a manicure or a pedicure to create beautiful, well-groomed nails. They need to be properly nourished to prevent hardening and flaking. This blend of base oils and essential oils penetrates your nails, strengthening the follicles and encouraging healthy growth.

3 tablespoons **avocado** oil

1½ tablespoons **borage** oil

1½ tablespoons evening **primrose** oil

20 drops **carrot seed** essential oil

10 drops **lavender** essential oil

6 drops **cypress** essential oil

6 drops **lemon** essential oil

6 drops **rosemary** essential oil

1 Combine the ingredients in a prepared container, seal tightly, and shake well.

2 Stored in a cool, dry place, this oil will keep for 6 months. Shake before using.

yield
This recipe makes approximately ⅓ cup oil.

to use
Apply a few drops daily to each nail, allow to soak in for 5 minutes, then rub in any unabsorbed oil.

Eucalyptus & Herb Cuticle Oil

Weekly, even daily, conditioning of cuticles goes a long way toward creating stronger, better-looking nails. But this isn't just for aesthetic effect. Regular conditioning with cuticle oil discourages hardening and cracking, and prevents nail fungus and other corrosive conditions.

❶ Combine the ingredients in a prepared container, seal tightly, and shake well.

❷ Stored in a cool, dark place, this conditioner will keep for 1 year. Shake before using.

¼ cup **jojoba**

15 drops **carrot seed** essential oil

15 drops **eucalyptus** essential oil

10 drops **peppermint** essential oil

10 drops **tea tree** essential oil

6 drops **oregano** essential oil

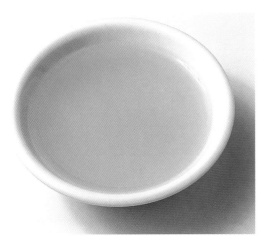

yield

This recipe makes approximately ¼ cup conditioner.

to use

Smooth a dab of conditioner onto each cuticle and nail once or twice a week.

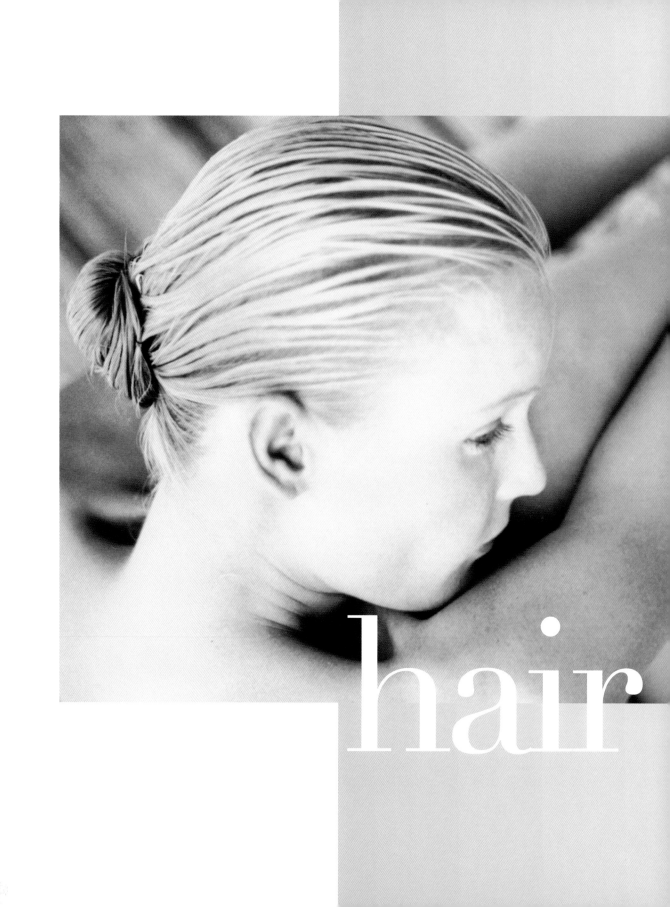

hair

When we are in good health, our hair looks lustrous and full of life. When we are sick or under stress, our hair appears languid and dull. Beautiful hair is a product of a balanced lifestyle; of course, good hair care is essential as well. Many commercial products strip hair of its natural protection by throwing off the proper pH balance, making hair either too dry or too oily.

The shampoos in this chapter will rid the scalp of any hair-care product residue and cleanse without eliminating the oils your follicles need for healthy growth. The rinses protect hair shafts against damage from toxins and bring out highlights. The deep treatments fortify damaged follicles and revitalize the scalp. All of this means that your hair will be as strong and healthy as it looks.

Use the recipes one at a time or in shampoo-rinse sequences as you see fit. Depending on the condition of your hair, you may treat it more or less frequently. Similarly, there are no fixed rules on when to add one of the deep treatments to your regimen. Indulge as often as your hair needs it, or perhaps in preparation for a special event. The result will be beautiful hair you can be proud of: soft, shining, and glowing with health and vitality.

In general, these shampoos won't produce the sort of intense lather you get from commercial products. Natural shampoos have a gentle, softly foaming lather that nevertheless thoroughly cleans your hair. The cosmetics industry would have us believe that it is lather that cleanses. It's not; it's ingredients like chamomile and citrus extracts that dissolve grease and clean the scalp.

Remember that the quantities given in the "to use" section are guidelines only. Unlike most commercial shampoos and conditioners, which are highly concen-trated and lather up with only one or two tablespoons, our hair products are unconcentrated. We generally suggest using about a quarter cup of shampoo and around one cup of rinse per treatment, depending upon your hair's length and thickness.

Because commercial products can tamper with hair's natural pH balance, you may find with natural products that your hair rediscovers its original properties: Straight hair becomes bouncier, and frizzy hair is much more manageable. These subtle changes are natural reactions to a toxin-free scalp.

hair

Basic Shampoo
with patchouli & geranium

You may find this hard to believe, but a good hair cleanser can be made without the numerous multisyllabic chemical compounds listed as ingredients on commercial shampoo labels. Castile soap, water, and a little sea salt are really all you need. Add a few drops of essential oil and you've got something special: a mild, effective shampoo suitable for all hair types that can be tailored to your whim. Here, we suggest a blend of two fragrant herbs—patchouli for its stimulating astringency and geranium for its ability to balance and regulate. You can change the scent of this basic shampoo by substituting (in the same quantities) the essential oils of lavender, rosemary, chamomile, sandalwood, sweet orange, or clary sage. Or choose one of our favorite blends of essential oils from the opposite page.

$^2/_3$ cup liquid **castile soap**

$^1/_3$ cup distilled **water**

$^1/_2$ teaspoon fine **sea salt**

12 drops **patchouli** essential oil

10 drops **geranium bourbon** essential oil

yield

This recipe makes approximately 1 cup, enough for 4 or 5 shampoos.

to use

Massage about ¼ cup of shampoo into wet hair, working to a lather. Rinse off with plenty of warm water.

❶ In a bowl, combine the castile soap and water and blend well. Stir in the salt and the essential oils.

❷ Transfer the shampoo to a prepared container and seal tightly. Stored in a cool, dark place, it will keep for 6 months. Shake before using.

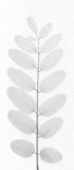

A musk-scented blend:

8 drops sandalwood essential oil

6 drops clary sage essential oil

6 drops cypress essential oil

4 drops lemongrass essential oil

A sweet-scented blend:

6 drops rose otto

6 drops sandalwood essential oil

4 drops jasmine absolute

4 drops patchouli essential oil

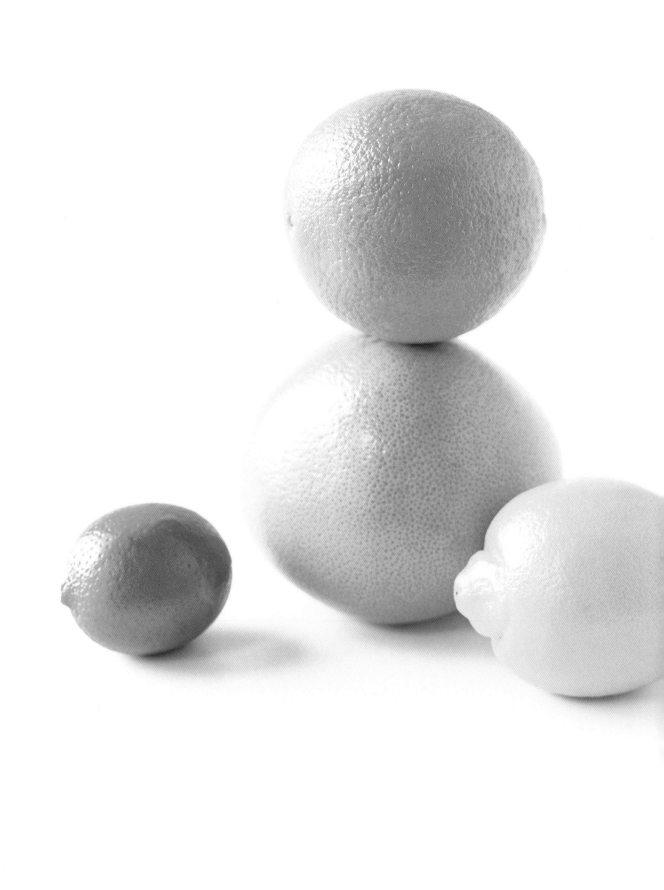

Sparkling Citrus Shampoo
for oily hair

Anyone with oily hair should try this shampoo. The acids in citrus essential oils act as mild solvents to gently dissolve oily buildup of grease and dirt and restore shine, while chamomile and rosemary condition follicles, improving balance and strengthening hair.

1. In a saucepan, bring the water to a boil, then remove from the heat. Add the chamomile and rosemary. Cover and let steep for 25 minutes. Strain off and discard the solids. Add the castile soap, sweet almond oil, lemon and sweet orange essential oils, and salt, and blend well. Cover and allow to cool to room temperature.

2. Transfer the shampoo to a prepared container and seal tightly. Stored in a refrigerator, it will keep for 2 weeks. Shake before using.

$\frac{1}{3}$ cup distilled **water**

2 tablespoons **chamomile** flowers

1 tablespoon **rosemary** leaves

$\frac{2}{3}$ cup liquid **castile soap**

2 teaspoons **sweet almond** oil

$\frac{1}{4}$ teaspoon **lemon** essential oil

$\frac{1}{4}$ teaspoon **sweet orange** essential oil

1 teaspoon fine **sea salt**

yield

This recipe makes approximately 1 cup, enough for 4 or 5 shampoos.

to use

Massage about ¼ cup of shampoo into wet hair, working to a lather. Rinse off with plenty of warm water.

Urban Herbal Hair Cleanser

City dwellers who confront smog, soot, and engine exhaust every day need a shampoo that is especially effective at cleaning away such gritty impurities. This shampoo provides high-powered cleansing but is mild enough that it won't dry out your locks, even with frequent use.

⅓ cup distilled **water**

1 teaspoon **lavender** leaves and flowers

1 teaspoon **nettle**

1 teaspoon **peppermint**

1 teaspoon **thyme**

⅔ cup liquid **castile soap**

1 teaspoon fine **sea salt**

1 teaspoon **sweet almond** oil

1 teaspoon **witch hazel** extract

6 drops **ylang-ylang** essential oil

4 drops **clary sage** essential oil

① In a saucepan, bring the water to a boil, then remove from the heat, and add in the lavender, nettle, peppermint, and thyme. Cover and let steep for 25 minutes. Strain off and discard the solids.

② Add the castile soap to the herb-infused water, followed by the salt, sweet almond oil, witch hazel, and the essential oils. Blend well, continuing to stir as the mixture cools and thickens.

③ When the mixture has reached room temperature, transfer it to a prepared container and seal tightly. Stored in a refrigerator, this shampoo will keep for 2 weeks. Shake before using.

yield

This recipe makes approximately 1 cup, enough for 4 or 5 shampoos.

to use

Massage about ¼ cup of cleanser into wet hair, working to a lather. Rinse off with plenty of warm water.

Chamomile & Egg Shampoo

Try this recipe for limp, lank hair that needs a little body. Egg protein returns life and bounce to your hair, while balancing chamomile ensures it a healthy shimmer. Not everyone's hair will respond to the egg, but if yours does, shampoo with it on three successive days at least once a month. Each time you do, your hair will absorb more protein.

1. In a bowl, combine the castor oil, grapefruit and lime juices, salt, and castile soap, and blend well. Gently whisk in the egg, the chamomile extract, and the essential oil.

2. Transfer the shampoo to a prepared container and seal tightly. Stored in a refrigerator, it will keep for 1 week. Shake before using.

1 teaspoon castor oil

1 teaspoon grapefruit juice

1 teaspoon lime juice

½ teaspoon fine sea salt

¾ cup liquid castile soap

1 lightly beaten egg

½ ounce chamomile extract

16 drops chamomile essential oil

yield

This recipe makes approximately 1 cup, enough for 4 or 5 shampoos.

to use

Massage about ¼ cup of shampoo into wet hair, working to a lather. Leave on for a few minutes to allow the egg proteins to penetrate the hair shafts. Rinse off with plenty of cool water (if it's too hot, the egg will start to cook).

Peppermint Shampoo

Here's a tingly scalp-cooling remedy for the dog days of summer. The trio of mints cleanses your hair and refreshes your spirit, while jojoba and wheat germ rehydrate hair shafts thirsty from exposure to the sun. This shampoo is great for all hair types, but the moisturizing action of the oils makes it especially beneficial for dry, brittle hair. If you can't find bergamot mint essential oil, substitute five extra drops of spearmint essential oil.

$^2/_3$ cup liquid castile soap

$^1/_3$ cup distilled water

2 teaspoons jojoba

1 teaspoon fine sea salt

1 teaspoon wheat germ oil

20 drops peppermint essential oil

5 drops spearmint essential oil

5 drops bergamot mint essential oil

❶ In a bowl, combine the castile soap and water and blend well. Stir in the remaining ingredients.

❷ Transfer the shampoo to a prepared bottle and cap tightly. Stored in a cool, dark place, it will keep for 2 weeks. Shake before using.

yield
This recipe makes approximately 1 cup, enough for 5 or 6 shampoos.

to use
Massage about ¼ cup of shampoo into wet hair, working to a lather. Rinse off with plenty of warm water.

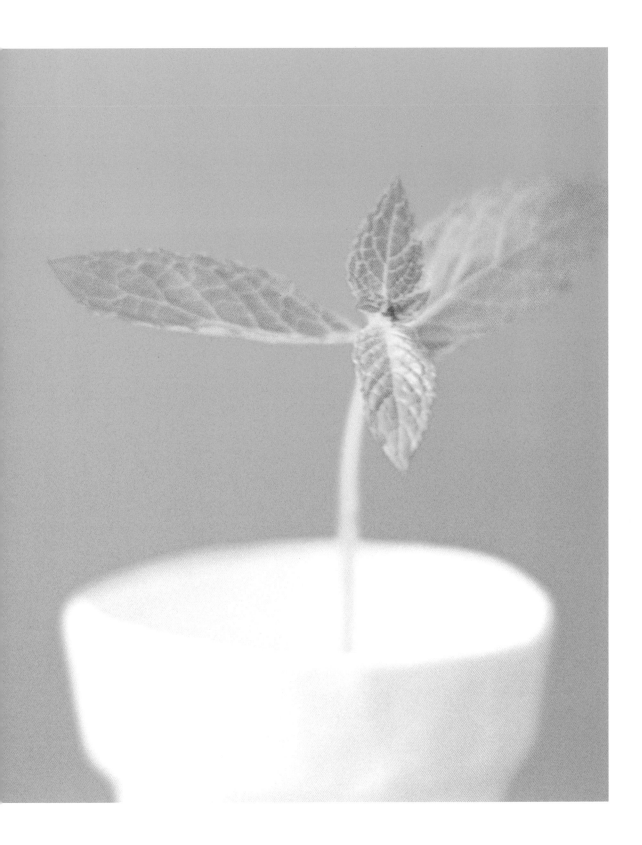

Chamomile & Rosemary Rinse

Every time you wash your hair, cleansing agents react with tap water to form protein and mineral deposits that accumulate on your follicles. Cut through that buildup with this easy-to-make vinegar treatment—its mild acidity and pleasant scent make for a nice, simple rinse.

4 **chamomile** tea bags

2 cups distilled **water**

¼ cup fresh **rosemary**

2 tablespoons **apple cider** vinegar

yield
This recipe makes enough for 1 rinse.

to use
After shampooing and rinsing with clean water, pour herbal rinse over wet hair and massage into scalp for a few minutes. Then rinse out with plenty of clean warm water.

❶ Open the chamomile tea bags and pour the herbs into a bowl. In a saucepan bring the water to a boil and pour over the chamomile. Add the fresh rosemary and let the mixture steep for 15 minutes.

❷ Add the apple cider vinegar. Strain off and discard the herbs. Use immediately.

Horsetail & Nettle Rinse
for dandruff control

While all types of hair will benefit from this excellent conditioning rinse, it is particularly useful for anyone with dandruff. The combination of silica-rich horsetail and nettle works synergistically to stimulate the scalp and improve hair strength. Any variety of mint—peppermint, spearmint, horsemint, or any of the several thousand subspecies—will have the same effect.

1. In a prepared container, combine the apple cider vinegar and the herbs, and seal tightly. Refrigerate for 2 weeks, to allow the herbs to steep into the vinegar.

2. Strain the vinegar into a bowl and discard the solids. Wash out the original container.

3. Return the rinse to the container and seal tightly. Stored in a refrigerator, it will keep for 6 months.

2 cups **apple cider** vinegar

1/2 cup **chamomile** flowers

1/2 cup **horsetail**

1/2 cup **mint**

1/2 cup **nettle**

yield

This recipe makes approximately 2 cups, enough for 8 to 10 rinses.

to use

After shampooing and towel-drying hair, rub 3 tablespoons of rinse into scalp and leave on for a few minutes. Then rinse out thoroughly. For best results, use this rinse at least twice a week.

Scalp-Stimulating Rinse

For centuries people have claimed that nettle, rosemary, and spearmint encourage hair growth. While there is no clinical evidence to prove the herbs actually promote growth or prevent hair loss, this fragrant blend will leave all types of hair soft, shiny, and easy to manage—and it may even make you believe that those old wives knew what they were talking about!

2 cups cold distilled **water**

1 cup **nettle**

1 cup **rosemary**

1 cup **spearmint**

1 **clove**

yield
This recipe makes approximately 2 cups, enough for 2 rinses.

to use
After shampooing and rinsing with clean water, pour 1 cup of rinse over wet hair. Catch the runoff as you pour and repeat several times. Do not rinse out.

❶ In a saucepan, over low heat, combine the ingredients and bring to a boil. Reduce the heat and simmer, uncovered, for 10 minutes. Remove from the heat, cover, and allow to steep until cooled to room temperature. Strain off and discard the solids.

❷ Transfer the rinse to a prepared container and seal tightly. Stored in a refrigerator, it will keep for 4 days.

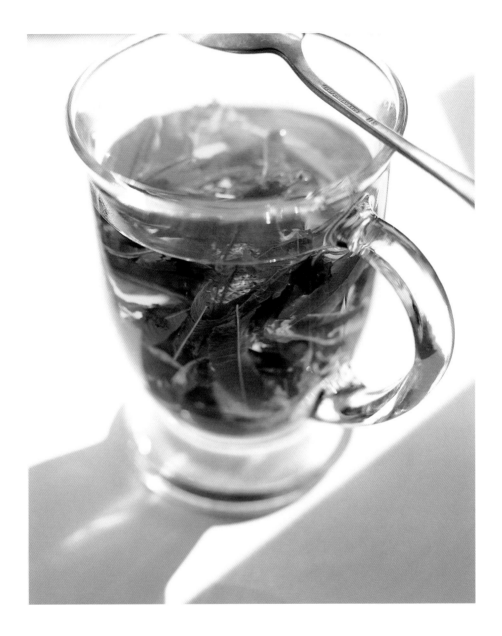

Apple Cider & Beer Rinse

The hops in beer relax frizz and improve shine. Vinegar strips away chemical build-up. Together, they complement each other beautifully—except for their scent. That problem is solved here with the addition of three essential oils, whose fragrances enhance hair with every shake of the head.

¼ cup **apple cider** vinegar

1 cup **beer**

20 drops **lemon** essential oil

20 drops **rosemary** essential oil

20 drops **sage** essential oil

1 Whisk all the ingredients together.

2 Use immediately.

yield

This recipe makes enough for 1 rinse.

to use

After shampooing and rinsing with clean water, pour herbal rinse over wet hair and massage into scalp for a few minutes. Then rinse out with plenty of warm water.

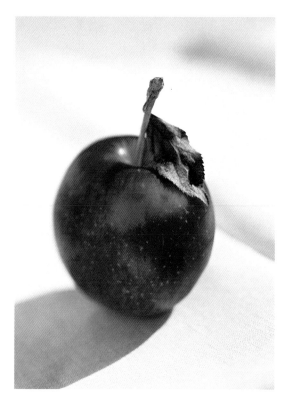

Granny's Herbal Hair Rinse

This rinse is amazingly beneficial to your hair and scalp. Anna's Granny insisted that everybody should use it at least once a week. In fact, she claimed she would have rinsed with it every day if only she'd had more time to comb the woods for the harder-to-find ingredients. Fortunately, you shouldn't have to resort to this: All of these herbs can be obtained at a good herb store, and it's worth seeking them out. In contrast to vinegar-based hair rinses, this rinse should not be washed out with water, but left in for the hair to get the maximum benefit.

① In a saucepan, combine the ingredients and bring to a boil. Remove from the heat, cover, and steep for 5 minutes. Strain, cover again, and allow to cool.

② Use as soon as the rinse is cool enough to pour on your scalp.

4 cups cold distilled **water**

¼ cup **birch** bark

¼ cup **chamomile** flowers

¼ cup **elderberry** flowers and leaves

¼ cup **horsetail**

¼ cup **nettle**

¼ cup **walnut** leaves

¼ cup **white oak** bark

¼ cup **yarrow** flowers

yield

This recipe makes enough for 1 rinse.

to use

Wet hair with one-third of the rinse. Then shampoo and rinse with clean water. Pour the remaining rinse over your hair and allowing it to penetrate for a few minutes. Then dry your hair as normal.

Rosemary & Cider Vinegar Rinse

One of the best conditioners you can use after a gentle herbal shampoo is a weak vinegar rinse. Infused with rosemary, which stimulates circulation, unclogs follicles, and deep-cleans pores, this one is simple and especially effective. Add a tablespoon of it to two cups of water and pour it over your hair as a final rinse. Better still, catch the runoff in a basin and repeat the rinse several times.

1 cup **rosemary**

2 cups **apple cider** vinegar

yield

This recipe makes approximately 2 cups, enough for 16 to 20 rinses.

to use

Add 1 tablespoon of rinse to 2 cups of water and pour over clean, wet hair. Catch the runoff and repeat. Do not rinse out.

1. In a prepared container, combine the rosemary and the apple cider vinegar and seal tightly.

2. Refrigerate for 7 to 10 days, to let the rosemary steep into the vinegar. Strain off and discard the solids.

3. Return the conditioner to the container and seal tightly. Stored in a refrigerator, it will keep for 3 months.

Chamomile & Tea Tree Conditioner

If your hair needs something a little more intensive than an herbal rinse, use this all-purpose oil-pack conditioner before shampooing. The base oils, jojoba and evening primrose, are restorative and nourishing, and help build up your hair's cell walls to make it look more alive. Chamomile and tea tree condition the scalp, prevent dandruff, and provide nutrients that moisturize and regulate oil secretion.

1 In a small bowl, combine ingredients and blend well.

2 Use immediately.

12 drops **chamomile** essential oil

10 drops **tea tree** essential oil

1 teaspoon evening **primrose** oil

1 teaspoon **jojoba**

8 drops **carrot seed** essential oil

6 drops **lavender** essential oil

yield

This recipe makes enough for 1 treatment.

to use

Massage the conditioner into dampened hair and scalp. Leave for 5 minutes or so, then wet hair without rinsing out all the conditioner. Follow by shampooing and rinsing with an herbal rinse suitable to your hair type.

Borage Conditioner
for fragile hair

Borage, known as the "herb of gladness," has a reputation for lifting the spirits and dispelling gloom. Certainly, its pretty blue flower, which blooms all summer long, is a heartwarming addition to any garden. In this treatment, the plant's oil has a similarly uplifting effect as it nurtures and strengthens fragile, damaged hair. When your hair needs some perking up use this conditioner before shampooing.

1 tablespoon **borage** oil

1 tablespoon **shea butter**

1 teaspoon **jojoba**

1 teaspoon liquid **lecithin**

1 teaspoon **sweet almond** oil

1/2 teaspoon evening **primrose** oil

20 drops **chamomile** essential oil

1 In the top of a double boiler, over low heat, combine all the ingredients except the chamomile essential oil. Heat gently until the shea butter is just melted and the lecithin has blended. Remove the mixture from the heat, cover, and cool to room temperature.

2 Stir in the chamomile essential oil. Use immediately.

yield
This recipe makes enough for 1 treatment.

to use
Work the conditioner into dampened hair and leave for about 10 minutes. Without rinsing, shampoo with a gentle herbal shampoo, and finish with an herbal rinse.

Essential Oil Conditioner

When you don't have time to brew an herbal hair conditioner, try this simple scalp-stimulating solution. All you have to do is mix together four essential oils in the palm of your hand and massage them through the hair. The conditioner immediately penetrates the hair shafts, leaving no oily residue. This recipe is geared for hair of medium length and thickness. Increase or decrease the number of drops depending upon the length and thickness of your hair.

1. In the palm of your hand, mix the oils together with your fingers.

2. Use immediately.

3 drops **carrot seed** essential oil

3 drops **chamomile** essential oil

3 drops **lavender** essential oil

3 drops **rosemary** essential oil

yield
This recipe makes enough for 1 treatment.

to use
After shampooing, towel-dry hair. Apply the conditioner by rubbing, brushing, or combing it into hair, starting at the ends (which need the most conditioning) and working to the scalp.

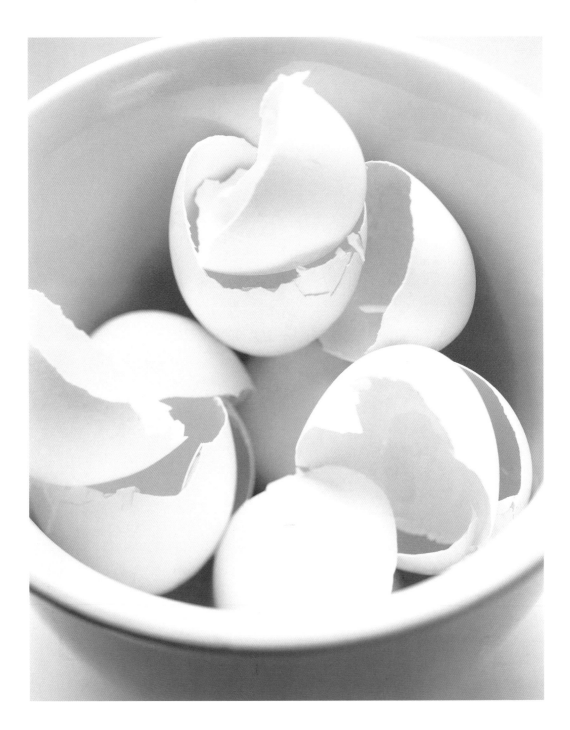

Egg Protein Conditioning Treatment

Beauty rest is not to be underestimated. Sometimes the best present you can give yourself is some quiet time. This treatment not only deeply conditions your hair. it forces you to put your feet up and relax for a while so you'll end up feeling as good as your hair will look.

1. In a mixing bowl, whisk the ingredients together until the honey is completely blended.

2. Use immediately.

2 eggs

3 tablespoons jojoba

2 tablespoons honey

1 tablespoon wheat germ oil

yield

This recipe makes enough for 1 treatment.

to use

Before shampooing, apply the conditioner to dampened hair, and wrap hair up in a towel for 45 minutes to 2 hours. Proceed with your normal regimen, making sure to rinse with cool water (if it's too hot, the egg will start to cook).

Yogurt & Egg Treatment
for flyaway hair

In the centuries before chemicals provided us with hairspray in aerosol canisters, people controlled dry, flyaway hair with this simple concoction, an intensive conditioning treatment that controls even the wildest hair by coating the shafts with proteins that both nourish and moisturize. The result is soft, shiny, manageable hair. Use this conditioner once every two weeks, or more frequently if your hair continues to insist on taking flight.

6 tablespoons plain **yogurt**

1 egg

yield
This recipe makes enough for 1 treatment.

to use
After shampooing, apply the conditioner and massage thoroughly into hair. Leave for about 10 minutes, then rinse out with cool water (if it's too hot, the egg will start to cook).

1 In a bowl, whisk the ingredients together until they are well blended.

2 Use immediately.

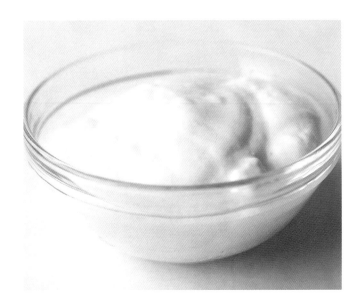

Herbal Clay Pack

Like a mud pack for the hair, this deep-cleaning, conditioning treatment will leave hair soft and glowing with health. The essential oil blend combines astringent and moisturizing properties to remove impurities from the hair follicles and promote strong growth.

1 In a bowl, whisk the ingredients together until the oils are fully incorporated.

2 Transfer the clay pack to a prepared container and seal tightly. Stored in the refrigerator, it will keep for 1 year.

$\frac{1}{4}$ cup **borage** oil

$\frac{1}{4}$ cup evening **primrose** oil

$\frac{1}{4}$ cup **jojoba**

$\frac{1}{4}$ cup **white clay**

20 drops **rosemary** essential oil

10 drops **cypress** essential oil

10 drops **lemon** essential oil

10 drops **sage** essential oil

6 drops **birch** essential oil

yield

This recipe makes approximately 1 cup, enough for 3 or 4 treatments.

to use

Pour ⅓ cup of clay pack onto dampened hair and work in, massaging the scalp as well. Then shampoo out, twice if necessary, and follow up with a conditioning rinse.

Hot Avocado Oil Treatment
for damaged hair

Sun, wind, rain, smoke, pollution, dust, life in general, even many commercial hair-care products: All can wreak havoc on your hair. For natural damage control, apply this oil treatment once a week before shampooing. It will strengthen your hair and leave it shining with vitality.

¼ avocado, mashed

3 tablespoons avocado oil

2 tablespoons jojoba

2 tablespoons lime juice

① In a small bowl, whisk the ingredients together, then warm them by placing the small bowl into a larger bowl filled halfway with hot water. Stir occasionally to distribute the heat evenly.

② As soon as the mixture is at body temperature, apply it to your damp hair.

yield

This recipe makes enough for 1 treatment.

to use

Apply directly to dampened hair, working from the scalp through the hair to the ends. Wrap your head in a warm damp towel (use an old towel, as the avocado may stain it). Leave the treatment on for about 20 minutes. Without rinsing, shampoo hair, then rinse thoroughly.

Sandalwood & Lavender Treatment Gel

Intensively moisturizing and nutritious, this is a gourmet restoration for the wildest head of hair. Sandalwood—serene, calming, and enriching—and soothing lavender are two of the most versatile and effective essential oils. Together with comfrey root and gelatin, they tame the frizziest mop and bring it to beauty.

1. In a small saucepan, bring the water to a boil and pour it over the chopped comfrey root in a bowl. Cover and let steep for 30 minutes. Strain off and discard the solids. Rinse the saucepan.

2. Pour the liquid back into the saucepan and bring to a boil, then remove from the heat. Add the gelatin, and stir to dissolve. Mix in the vinegar and the essential oils. Cover the mixture and let cool to room temperature.

3. Use immediately.

$^1/_2$ cup distilled **water**

$^1/_4$ cup chopped **comfrey** root

2 tablespoons **gelatin**

1 teaspoon **apple cider** vinegar

10 drops **sandalwood** essential oil

6 drops **carrot seed** essential oil

4 drops **chamomile** essential oil

4 drops **clary sage** essential oil

4 drops **lavender** essential oil

yield

This recipe makes enough for 1 treatment.

to use

Work the gel through hair, making sure your whole head is covered. Leave for 15 minutes or so. Then rinse thoroughly, and shampoo. Repeat every 7 to 10 days for best results.

Glossary

Unless otherwise noted, the following ingredients are available at natural food markets or herb stores. Mail order sources for essential oils and other supplies are listed on pages 140-41.

Alcohol *See* Grain alcohol.

Almond oil (or sweet almond oil) moisturizes and helps prevent loss of moisture from the skin. Mild, very soothing, and easily absorbed, it is used in massage oils, hand creams, body milks, and night creams.

Almonds are emollient and, when finely ground, gently abrasive, which make them effective in cleansing scrubs and exfoliants.

Aloe vera gel, the watery substance inside the aloe leaf, is moisturizing and soothing for a variety of skin discomforts. Fresh aloe gel is the best; you can grow your own aloe vera plants or buy the leaves in a natural food market. Slit them down the side and gently scrape the gel out of the leaf. When buying aloe, look for gel that is at least 99% pure, with no additives; gels that look thick are probably chemically based.
Warning: Can be an irritant; perform a skin patch test before using.

Aloe vera oil has the same healing properties as aloe vera gel, but has a consistency that is better suited to creams and lotions.
Warning: Can be an irritant; perform a skin patch test before using.

Amber resin, formed by the sap of Indian amber trees, gives preparations an exotically sweet, almost candy-like aroma. Long known as a skin-softening agent, it is an excellent addition to creams and lotions. It is sold in chunks by the gram in herb shops, incense shops, and fragrance stores.

Apple is a natural source of malic acid and vitamin C, both of which dissolve facial grease and dirt.

Apple cider vinegar diluted with distilled water is gently astringent and soothing to itchy, dry skin. It also helps to restore the skin's natural pH level. In hair products, it works as a mild solvent to help prevent soap scum buildup.
Warning: Can be an irritant; perform a skin patch test before using.

Avocado, rich in vitamin E, is a superior nutrient for skin.

Avocado oil is especially beneficial in preparations for very dry skin. It has outstanding moisturizing and regenerative properties, and is also a good hair-growth stimulant.

Baking soda possesses skin-softening and -soothing qualities in water-based solutions. It is used as a disinfectant in foot powders, as a mild abrasive in tooth powders, and as a softener in bath salts.

Basil essential oil, distilled from the herb, has an aroma both spicy and floral, and is antibacterial by nature. In aromatherapy, it is said to be energizing, strengthening, and refreshing.
Warning: Avoid when pregnant.

Bay (or sweet bay, bay laurel) is an astringent, antiseptic, and fragrant herb. In aromatherapy, it is believed to build confidence and improve mood.

Bay essential oil (or laurel leaf) acts as a local antiseptic and a treatment for dandruff and dry or irritated skin. In aromatherapy, it is said to be relaxing.
Warning: Avoid prolonged exposure to the sun after application.

Beer's gaseous bubbles act as gentle solvents in hair rinses, eliminating dirt and excess oil. The hops work to relax frizz and improve shine.

Beeswax, grated and melted, is an emulsifying wax that softens and protects skin without clogging pores. It is available at craft supply stores in addition to natural food markets and herb stores.
Warning: Can be an irritant; perform a skin patch test before using.

Bergamot essential oil is distilled from the fruit of a citrus tree grown in the Mediterranean. Its fruity, floral scent — spicier than that of most citrus oils — enhances aromatic blends. In aromatherapy, it is considered uplifting and confidence-building.

Bergamot mint essential oil, which is unrelated to bergamot essential oil, is a member of the mint family. It has a sweet, mild aroma that can be substituted for spearmint essential oil.

Birch bark was relied upon by Native Americans for treating all sorts of skin conditions. It contains a small quantity of a substance that is commonly included in acne medications and is found in preparations for problem skin.

Birch (or sweet birch) essential oil has a sweet, wintergreen-like fragrance. The oil contains methyl salicylate, which has counterirritant and analgesic properties. Use it in minute quantities, as suggested in the recipes.

Borage, a leafy herb with a small, blue, star-shaped flower, helps promote healthy cell growth in sensitive, dry skin.

Borage oil is often recommended for skin treatments. It can help heal sun-damaged skin, prevent wrinkles, combat dehydration, and maintain elasticity. It is also a good moisturizer for dry or permed hair.

Borax (or borax powder) is a white crystalline mineral powder that is commonly combined with beeswax to act as an emulsifying agent and water softener. Although prolonged exposure to full-strength borax can cause skin irritation, it is considered completely safe in the small quantities called for in these recipes. It is available in the laundry section of supermarkets, or at pharmacies.
Warning: Can be an irritant; perform a skin patch test before using.

Buttermilk acts as an emollient in cleansing milks for dry skin. It is available at most supermarkets.

Cajeput essential oil, which comes from the Australian or Southeast Asian cajeput tree, a member of the myrtle family, is similar to, but less potent than, tea tree oil and can be substituted for tea tree oil. Its manifold healing properties include relieving pain and soothing skin irritations.
Warning: Avoid prolonged exposure to the sun after application.

Calendula flowers, also known as field and pot marigolds, soothe and heal rough, dry, cracked skin, especially in cases of eczema, sunburn, and inflammation. The petals are astringent, antiseptic, and antifungal.

Carrot seed essential oil produces a spicy-sweet aroma in natural perfumes and skin-care products. The oil is good for cleansing, toning, and stimulating skin elasticity, and is also helpful in treating dermatitis, eczema, sensitive skin, and wrinkles. In aromatherapy, it is considered renewing, nourishing, and restoring.

Castile soap, generally made from olive and vegetable oils, is a multipurpose cleanser for bathing and shampooing. It can be store-bought or made at home following the recipe included in the book COUNTRY LIVING HANDMADE SOAP.

Castor oil, the thick, viscous oil of castor plant seeds, tempers skin problems, conditions hair, and stimulates the scalp. It also works *as* a moisturizer in sun oils, bath oils, lip balms, and face products for all but very oily skin.

Cedarwood essential oil, which is naturally antiseptic, has a long history of treating skin afflictions. Its woodsy, balsam-like aroma adds substance and a friendly note to any perfume blend. In aromatherapy, it is considered settling, comforting, mentally empowering, and calming.

Chamomile is a mildly fragrant skin-softening herb that many people regard as a cure-all. It has astringent, healing, and anti-inflammatory properties. The oil infusions help heal eczema, insect bites, and minor wounds. The water infusions deep-clean pores. When powdered, chamomile mixes well and adds fragrance to bath sachets and body powders.
Warning: May cause allergic reaction in hay fever sufferers.

Chamomile essential oil has a sweet, fruity aroma that adds soothing warmth to massage oils, shampoos, and all kinds of herbal skin preparations.
Warning: Can be an irritant; dilute well and perform a skin patch test before using.

Chamomile extract is an extraction of chamomile flowers, alcohol, and water. In creams and lotions it acts as an emollient, soothing and clarifying skin.

Cinnamon, a spice that comes from the inner bark of any of several trees of the laurel family that grow throughout Africa and Asia, has astringent and anti-bacterial properties. It is used as a flavoring in tooth powders and mouthwashes.

Clary sage essential oil, distilled from the flowering tops of the clary sage plant, gives off a balsam-like scent that blends well with other botanicals. In aromatherapy, it is considered focusing, euphoric, and an aid to visualization.
Warning: Avoid when pregnant.

Clove is a spice that functions as an antibacterial agent in tooth powders and mouthwashes.

Clove essential oil possesses antibacterial properties that make it effective in mouthwashes.
Warning: Can be an irritant; dilute well and perform a skin patch test before using. Avoid when pregnant.

Cocoa butter comes from the bean of the cocoa plant. The rich source of skin-softening nutrients is included in preparations for skin maintenance, moisturizing, and repair. Though solid at room temperature, cocoa butter melts quickly on your skin.
Warning: Can be an irritant; perform a skin patch test before using.

Coconut oil softens and moisturizes. It is added to sun products and foam baths to make the skin supple, and to conditioners for damaged hair, body oils for dry skin, creams for sensitive skin, and lip balms for cracked lips.

Comfrey is an herb whose roots and leaves contain a healing compound called allantoin that, when added to creams or lotions or infused in olive oil, creates a topical remedy for all types of skin afflictions. It is available in bulk from most herb suppliers.

Cornmeal, or finely ground dried corn, is added to facial masks to absorb excess oil, and to scrubs as a gentle exfoliant.

Cream, an emollient, works in cleansing milks and other facial and body scrub preparations as a remedy for dry skin.

Cucumber makes a mild, healing cleanser and a soothing toner for alleviating inflammations and irritations of the skin.

Cypress essential oil is distilled from the leaves and twigs of the cypress tree. It has a refreshing, spicy, piney aroma that hints of evergreen needles. Its astringent, antiseptic, and sedative properties can help ease nervous tension and heal wounds. In aromatherapy, it is thought to be purifying and balancing.

Dill essential oil, distilled from the herb, has a pungent aroma that adds distinction to cleansing, bathing, and toning products.

Distilled water has been purified by a sequence of evaporation and condensation.

Egg, especially egg yolk, is useful in masks and hair preparations since it contains protein and trace amounts of lecithin, an emulsifier that is a natural component of our own hair and skin.

Elderberry flowers help fade freckles, smooth wrinkles, soothe sunburn, and soften skin and hair.

Emulsifying wax is one of the best and most stable emulsifiers to pair with herbal ingredients in creams or lotions. It generally consists of vegetable or botan-ically based oils such as rice bran and is usually sold under a house brand name by cosmetic suppliers. Do not substitute "emulsifying ointment."

Epsom salts are pure mineral salts for softening both water and skin.

Eucalyptus tree leaves have a powerful earthy aroma and contain compounds that make them good natural muscle relaxants and respiratory stimulants.

Eucalyptus essential oil is popular because of its wonderful aroma and antiseptic, antibacterial, and antiviral properties. Helpful for acne, it is mildly stimulating and may create a gentle tingle as it increases circulation to the skin and hair follicles.

Evening primrose oil comes from the leaves, seeds, and roots of the evening primrose flower. It is rich in gamma-lineolenic acid, which helps maintain skin elastic-ity. Its moisturizing, nourishing, and antiaging properties are effective in antiwrinkle eye creams, hand creams, lip balms, and preparations for mature skin.

Fennel (or sweet fennel) essential oil, from the leaves, seeds, and stems of the fennel herb, has a spicy, sweet aroma that gives a sharp note to the fragrance of a preparation. In aromatherapy, it is an emotional restorative because it is warming and invigorating.

Fennel seeds have a balsam-like fragrance and antiseptic properties when ground or finely chopped.

Fir needle essential oil, distilled from the pointy needles and rough stems of fir trees, has a fresh, green, spicy scent. In soaps and, in minute quantities, in body oils it refreshes, centers, and harmonizes aromatherapeutic properties.
Warning: Can be an irritant; dilute well and perform a skin patch test before using.

Gelatin, a binding agent derived from animal proteins, is used solely for its gelling properties.

Geranium is a common floral herb, the leaves of which are mildly astringent.

Geranium bourbon essential oil has a powerful, leafy, somewhat green aroma that is sweet with minty undertones. It is included in skin-care products for its cleansing, astringent, and antiseptic properties. In aromatherapy, it is considered balancing and centering.
Warning: Avoid when pregnant.

Ginger essential oil has the aromatic and healing properties of ginger, which has long been regarded as a powerful general tonic, especially in Asian cultures.

Glycerin, a liquid vegetable-based derivative of soap, moistens and protects the skin, soothing inflammations. It also acts as a humectant, drawing moisture out of the air into the skin.
Warning: Can be an irritant; perform a skin patch test before using.

Glycerin soap is more refined and contains more glycerin than regular vegetable-based soaps.

Grain alcohol has been distilled from grain, and is considered the best for botanical extracts and tinctures. It is generally available in liquor stores as Everclear. If unavailable, substitute vodka.

Grapefruit essential oil has a strong citrus aroma. It tones and firms the skin, and has most of the qualities of other citrus essential oils (*see* lime, lemon, and sweet orange). In aromatherapy, it is said to be refreshing, balancing, and uplifting.
Warning: Avoid prolonged exposure to the sun after application.

Grapefruit juice is a natural skin toner that works alone or in combination with other fruit juices.

Green clay is finely powdered cosmetic clay, used in facial masks for its ability to draw impurities out of the skin, tighten pores, and absorb oils. It is available at cosmetics supply shops.

Honey is an emollient that soothes the skin and protects it with an extremely thin film when added to creams, lotions, and lip balms. If possible, choose raw honey, preferably straight from the comb, as it is less processed and more pure.

Honeysuckle flowers relax muscles and soothing skin irritations.

Horsetail is a ferny herb rich in silica, which makes it gently abrasive and therefore good for removing dirt and grime from the skin and hair.

Jasmine absolute is a highly concentrated alcohol extraction (not an essential oil) made from the jasmine flower. It has a powerful fragrance and is good for moisturizing aging and sensitive skin. Indole, a natural component of jasmine, is believed to be similar to the chemical in humans that is said to stimulate physical attraction, so jasmine is included in many perfumes. Pure absolute is best, but the more available and less costly diluted variety works, too.

Jojoba, the oil pressed from the seeds of the jojoba plant, is rich in proteins and moisturizing properties. It stimulates and conditions the hair, making it smooth and shiny; soothes and eliminates skin problems; and protects against premature wrinkling. Jojoba is found in treatments for permed, dyed, gray, damaged, and delicate hair, and in nourishing hand and facial-care products.

Juniper essential oil, from the berries, leaves, and wood of the juniper shrub, has a piney, woodsy, balsam-like aroma, and is a particular favorite in masculine fragrance blends. In aromatherapy, it is thought to be restoring, strength-ening, and refreshing.
Warning: Avoid when pregnant.

Lavender's aptitude for cleansing and beautifying the skin is reflected in its name, which comes from the Latin verb "to wash." This purple flowering herb also has numerous healing properties, including relieving skin inflammations and sunburns, and is generally considered balancing, soothing, gently clarifying, and normalizing for the skin.

Lavender essential oil is made from the flowering tops of the lavender plant. It is known to be antiviral, antibiotic, antiseptic, and antifungal, and is repellent to mosquitoes and houseflies. In aromatherapy, it is believed to soothe nervous tension, insomnia, and depression.

Lavender water, a by-product of essential oil production, is a soothing and gentle toner with a relaxing aroma. It makes an fragrant addition to the water portion of recipes for creams and lotions.

Lecithin, one of nature's best emulsifiers, is derived from soybean oil. It comes in three forms: as a capsule, in bulk as a light brown granule, and as a gooey, dark reddish-brown substance known as liquid lecithin.

Lemon essential oil contains the essence of the rinds of some three dozen lemons for each half ounce of oil. It is a soothing disinfectant. In aromatherapy, it is considered energizing, uplifting, and renewing.
Warning: Can be an irritant; dilute well and perform a skin patch test before using. Avoid prolonged exposure to the sun after application.

Lemon juice, like other citrus juices, is an astringent, included in facial cleansers for its ability to naturally dissolve makeup and surface grime.

Lemongrass is an antibacterial, antifungal tropical grass that stimulates perspiration, which aids in detoxification, and relaxes muscles.

Lemongrass essential oil is derived from the long, pungent leaves of lemongrass. In skin-care preparations it is valued for its toning and mild disinfecting properties. In aromatherapy, a strong lemon scent is said to be calming, uplifting, and balancing.
Warning: Can be an irritant; dilute well and perform a skin patch test before using.

Lime essential oil in beauty treatments purifies and disinfects the skin. It also helps reduce the appearance of cellulite deposits. In aromatherapy, it is believed to relieve fatigue, elevate mood, energize, and refresh.
Warning: Avoid prolonged exposure to the sun after application.

Lime juice is mildly acidic, and works as an antioxidant and astringent in skin-care products.

Linden flower, from the linden tree, is added to bath preparations for its skin-softening properties.

Loofah, a gourd with flesh that is hard and brittle when dry yet soft and pleasantly scrubby when wet, can be used whole as an exfoliating sponge or finely ground as part of a facial scrub.

Marjoram essential oil, distilled from the oregano-like herb, is antiseptic, mildly disinfectant, calming to the body, and relaxing to the muscles. It has a sweet, mild, and spicy aroma, and is relied on in aromatherapy for purifying, cleansing, and warming.
Warning: Avoid when pregnant.

Milk, especially cow's milk, is a gentle emollient and wetting agent in cleansing milks, and also acts as an emulsifier.

Mint, specifically the spearmint and peppermint varieties, has a refreshing fragrance as well as astringent and antiseptic properties that make it popular in a wide range of preparations such as toners, mouthwashes, rinses, and balms.

Neroli essential oil, which is distilled from the flowers of the bitter orange tree, has a refreshing, spicy aroma that works especially well in rubbing oils, skin creams, and bath oils. In aromatherapy, it is considered soothing, exotic, and sensual.
Warning: Avoid prolonged exposure to the sun after application.

Nettle is an astringent herb with a stimulating and therapeutic effect on hair and skin. It is particularly well-suited for cleansing oily skin and nourishing damaged hair.

Oats (or rolled oats) have a high silica content, making them abrasive and mineral-rich, and when applied externally are considered beneficial for various skin conditions. Their exfoliating properties help masks and scrubs perform.

Olive oil, an all-around emollient, helps reduce wrinkles and replenish moisture and nutrients lost through exposure to the sun. It can be substituted for other base oils in most recipes. Extra-virgin olive oil, the oil from the first pressing of the olive, is the freshest, least acidic, and therefore most desirable variety for skin and hair preparations.

Orange essential oil *See* Sweet orange essential oil.
Warning: Avoid when pregnant. Avoid prolonged exposure to the sun after application.

Orange floral water, a by-product of the distillation of orange blossoms, is mildly antiseptic, astringent, and anti-inflammatory. Its aroma adds an uplifting note to creams and lotions.

Orange flowers and leaves are sweetly aromatic and said to reduce muscle tension and skin irritations.

Orange peel, when dried and ground, has mild antiseptic and abrasive properties that make it effective in facial preparations such as scrubs and masks.

Oregano essential oil, distilled from the herb, is a mild disinfectant with a green, herbaceous, spicy aroma that in aromatherapy invigorates and strengthens.

Palm stearic acid, a waxy substance derived from palm trees, thickens and stabilizes lotions and other beauty preparations, giving them a creamy, pearlescent quality. It is available in pharmacies, herb shops, candle supply stores, and by mail order.
Warning: Can be an irritant; perform a skin patch test before using.

Palma rosa essential oil, distilled from the palma rosa plant, has a sweet aroma as well as healing, regenerating, and moisturizing properties. In aromatherapy, it is described as mood-elevating, pain-relieving, and relaxing to the muscles.
Warning: Avoid when pregnant.

Parsley, the sturdy herb that often appears as a food garnish, contains numerous vitamins and minerals, as well as antibacterial properties that can help fight the germs that cause bad breath. When infused, it also possesses toning and firming qualities.

Patchouli, an herbal bush that grows in Indonesia, China, and Madagascar, is astringent, antiseptic, anti-inflammatory, and antifungal, but it is best known for its strong woodsy aroma.

Patchouli essential oil, a thick, dark, yellowish oil distilled from patchouli leaves, has long been highly esteemed by both medicinal herbalists and perfumers. For centuries it has been used as an insecticide and as a remedy for acne, skin fungi, eczema, and dandruff. Its scent is said to be romantic, sensual, and stimulating.

Peppermint, a mildly antiseptic herb, soothes itchy, dry, or burned skin. *See* Mint.

Peppermint essential oil stimulates the skin with a tingling sensation. Because of its antiseptic nature, it is popular in a wide range of beauty preparations. In aromatherapy, it is considered invigorating, refreshing, and cooling.
Warning: Avoid when pregnant. Can be an irritant; dilute well and perform a skin patch test before using. Avoid prolonged exposure to the sun after application.

Queen Anne's lace is an aromatic flowering herb that soothes itchy, irritated skin.

Rolled oats *See* Oats.

Raspberry leaves are mildly astringent and anti-inflammatory. Added to creams, lotions, and bath preparations, they aid in soothing and softening the skin.

Rose geranium essential oil, a distillation made from the petals and stems of the rose geranium plant, is interchangeable with geranium bourbon essential oil. *See* Geranium bourbon essential oil.

Rose otto (or rose essential oil) is a highly concentrated oil produced from rose petals. (It takes some thirty rose petals for every one drop.) In skin creams, powders, and lotions, its antiseptic qualities treat dry, aging, and sensitive skin. Rose otto has a sweet, deep, long-lasting aroma that is said to be uplifting. Adding a drop to any hair, facial, or bath oil creates a luxurious, soothing experience. In aromatherapy, it is thought to be romantic, creative, directing, cheering, enchanting, and quixotic. Rose absolute, a highly concentrated alcohol extract — rather than an essential oil — is an economical alternative.
Warning: Avoid when pregnant.

Rose petals work as mild, soothing cleansers and skin softeners in bath salts, oils, and gels. *See* Rose otto and Rose water.

Rose water is a by-product of the distillation of rose petals for various rose essential oils. It brings a lovely aroma to all kinds of beauty-care products and is an emollient that is especially beneficial for dry, sensitive, and aging skin.

Rosemary's green, needle-like leaves contain many healing and cleansing properties and have a pungent, earthy aroma. For centuries, Europeans have believed that the herb stimulates hair growth.
Warning: Avoid if you have high blood pressure or epilepsy.

Rosemary essential oil stimulates blood flow and in turn endows the skin with a healthy pinkish glow. It is a general detoxifier in beauty treatments and is used in shampoos and conditioners to stimulate hair growth. In aromatherapy, it is considered warming, invigorating, and clarifying.

Warning: Avoid when pregnant or if you have high blood pressure or epilepsy.

Rosemary vinegar is created by infusing any vinegar with fresh or dried rosemary leaves, thus adding the herbs's deep-cleansing and stimulating power to vinegar's naturally astringent quality. It is included in hair rinses for its stimulating, nourishing properties.

Warning: Can be an irritant; perform a skin patch test before using.

Rosewood essential oil, distilled from the wood of the Brazilian rosewood tree, has a spicy yet freshly sweet scent that brightens up the aroma of many soaps, lotions, and massage oils. In aromatherapy, it is regarded as gently strengthening and relaxing. It is unrelated to the rose flower.

Safflower oil, a base oil with a smooth texture and a relatively high percentage of vitamin E, has almost no aroma or color, making it ideal for lotions with scented ingredients.

Sage's stimulating, mildly astringent blossoms and silver-green leaves are especially beneficial in skin cleansing, reducing large pores, eliminating dandruff, and highlighting color in graying hair.

Warning: Avoid if you have high blood pressure or epilepsy.

Sage essential oil, which has a slight undertone of camphor in its aroma, is astringent, anti-bacterial, and antibiotic. Added to facial preparations, it enhances stimulation and helps balance and tone blemish-prone skin.

Warning: Avoid when pregnant or if you have high blood pressure or epilepsy.

Salt softens water and helps relieve itchy skin. Most salts—from coarse kosher salts to various grades of sea salts to Epsom salts, which contain lots of trace minerals—are softening agents, cleansers, and exfoliators.

Sandalwood essential oil, distilled from the heartwood and roots of the sandalwood tree, blends well with other oils. Its mild, nutritive action makes it suitable for all skin types, but especially beneficial for dry, chapped, rashy, or inflamed skin conditions. In aromatherapy, it is thought to be relaxing, centering, and exotic.

Sea salt *See* Salt.

Shea butter, produced from the nut of the karite tree, is a moisturizer for the skin and hair. It softens, protects against dryness, prevents sun damage, and may help reduce stretch marks. It does, however, have a strong aroma that some people find off-putting.

Spearmint essential oil has a refreshing, cooling effect in mouthwashes and bathwater, and is considered energizing to the mind and body. In aromatherapy, it is said to be revitalizing.

Spearmint *See* Mint.

Spruce essential oil comes from the needles of the spruce tree and produces a sweet, pine-like, woodsy aroma that in aromatherapy is said to calm and encourage.

Star anise, the star-shaped herb that flavors licorice, serves as a mild antiseptic in various skin preparations and mouthwashes.

Sweet almond oil *See* Almond oil.

Sweet birch essential oil *See* Birch essential oil.

Sweet orange essential oil, pressed from the peel of sweet oranges, is a natural source of alpha-hydroxy acids, which gently exfoliate and encourage healthy new cell growth.

Warning: Avoid prolonged exposure to the sun after application.

Tangerine essential oil (or mandarine) is a gentle exfoliator. In aromatherapy, it relieves tension and depression.

Warning: Avoid when pregnant. Avoid prolonged exposure to the sun after application.

Tea tree essential oil is a medicinal-smelling, clear, colorless oil produced from leaves and twigs of the Australian *melaleuca alternifolia* plant. Its antifungal, antiseptic, antibiotic, and antiviral properties are helpful in treating all kinds of skin problems. If tea tree essential oil is unavailable, the similar but less potent cajeput essential oil makes a good substitute.

Warning: Can be an irritant; dilute well and perform a skin patch test before using.

Thyme leaves, with strong astringent, antiseptic, anti-bacterial, and stimulating properties, are added to a wide range of beauty products, from deodorants and balms to cleansers.

Warning: Avoid when pregnant or if you have high blood pressure.

Thyme essential oil, like the leaves from which it is derived, is astringent, antiseptic, and antibacterial. It has an intense, spicy aroma and should be used in small quantites only.

Warning: Avoid when pregnant or if you have high blood pressure.

Tomato, which absorbs easily into the skin, is rich in riboflavin and vitamins A and C, making it a nourishing addition to deep-treatment masks.

Valerian essential oil comes from the flowering valerian plant. It has an earthy, mossy scent and sedative, warming qualities that relieve skin irritations.

Vitamin E has a rejuvenating effect on the skin, including healing cuts and minimizing scarring. Natural sources of vitamin E include cold-pressed safflower, sunflower, and wheat germ oils. Use only the d-alpha tocopheryl vitamin E that is available in capsule or liquid form at natural food markets and pharmacies.

Warning: Can be an irritant; perform a skin patch test before using.

Walnut leaves are healing to the skin and are believed to help prevent hair loss.

Wheat germ oil helps prevent moisture loss and sun damage by keeping the skin well moisturized and conditioned. It is a good ingredient for healing damaged hair and skin because of its high concentration of vitamin E.

White clay is a finely powdered cosmetic clay that acts as an astringent in cosmetics and facial masks.

White cornmeal *See* Cornmeal.

White oak bark, when infused, is mildly astringent, soothing, and healing.

White willow bark is an astringent with cooling properties that help reduce inflammation.

Witch hazel bark *See* Witch hazel extract.

Witch hazel extract is made from the leaves, twigs, and bark of the deciduous witch hazel shrub or small tree. It has astringent properties that aid toners and clarifying lotions in tightening pores and reducing inflammations. The common witch hazel preparations found in pharmacies and grocery stores should be avoided as they often contain isopropyl (or rubbing) alcohol, which can be damaging to the skin. Use only the grain alcohol and water extract version sold in natural beauty product shops and natural food markets.

Yarrow flowers' emollient and anti-inflammatory properties treat many skin conditions. Available in bulk as a tea.

Yogurt, which contains beneficial enzymes from the bacterial cultures that turn milk into yogurt, is soothing to the skin and helpful in restoring its natural pH balance. Plain, natural, unpasturized yogurt with active cultures is the best for facial preparations.

Ylang-ylang essential oil comes from the ylang-ylang plant, a broad-leafed evergreen tropical shrub. It has a richly floral, jasmine-like aroma and toning properties that stimulate the skin to produce oil and regulate its natural oil balance.

Ingredients & Supplies

A Woman of Uncommon Scents
P.O. Box 103
Roxbury, PA 17251
(800) 377-3685
website:www.ecomall.com/biz/awscents
Essential oils

Ambrosia Natural Products
12 Colorado Ave.
Pueblo, CO 81004
(800) 887-5562
fax: (719) 595-0669
e-mail: norm@ambrosia-online.com
website: www.ambrosia-online.com
Essential oils

Aroma Terra
P.O. Box 83027
Phoenix, AZ 85071
(602) 371-4676
fax: (602) 371-4672
Amber, base and essential oils, bottles and jars, glycerin, herbs

Aroma Vera
5901 Rodeo Rd.
Los Angeles, CA 90016-4312
(800) 669-9514 or (310) 280-0407
fax: (310) 280-0395
Base and essential oils, bottles and jars

Aunt Mert's Cornmeal
P.O. Box 3416
Boone, NC 28607
(828) 297-4002
Stone-ground cornmeal

The Boston Jojoba Co.
P.O. Box 771
Middleton, MA 01949
(800) 256-5622
fax: (508) 777-9332
Jojoba

C-H Imports
P.O. Box 18411
Greensboro, NC 27419
(336) 282-9734
fax: (336) 288-3375
e-mail: bollini@msn.com
Essential oils, floral waters

Cleveland Bottle and Supply
(216) 881-3330
e-mail: bottle@ncweb.com
website: www.ncweb.com/biz/bottle
Bottles and jars, labeling supplies

Consolidated Plastics Co., Inc.
8181 Darrow Rd.
Twins Burge, OH 44087
(800) 362-1000
fax: (216) 425-3333
Bottles and jars, spatulas

Creation Herbal Products
P.O. Box 344
Deep Gap, NC 28618
(828) 262-0006
fax: (828) 262-1178
e-mail: creationsoap@boone.net
website: www.creationherbal.com
Base and essential oils, beeswax, herbs and herbal extracts, floral waters, glycerin soap, jojoba, rose water, vitamin E

Elk Mountain Herbs
214 Ord St.
Laramie, WY 82070
(888) 214-0404
website:www.wyomingwideweb/ElkMountainHerbs
Herbs and herbal extracts

Garden Past
P.O. Box 336130
Greenly, CO 80633
(970) 392-9704
Base and essential oils, herbs, bottles and jars, labeling supplies

Good Food
4960 Horseshoe Pike
Honeybrook, PA 19344
(800) 327-4406 or (610) 273-3776
fax: (610) 273-7652
e-mail: goodfood@goldenbarrel.com
Base oils

Harlan Fairbanks Co. Ltd.
12031 No. 5 Rd.
Richmond, BC V7A 4E9 Canada
(604) 275-8445
Base oils

Herb Garden
P.O. Box 9
Shipshewana, IN 46565
(800) 831-0504
Herbs

Herbal Accents
560 North Highway 101, Ste. 4A
Encinitas, CA 92024
(888) 440-4380 or (760) 633-4255
fax: (760) 632-7279
e-mail: Herbalacce@aol.com
website: www.member.aol.herbalacce
Base and essential oils, beeswax, clays, cocoa butter, glycerin, sea salt, shea butter, soap molds, vitamin E

Indiana Botanical Gardens
3401 West Thirty-Seventh Ave.
Hobart, IN 46342
(219) 947-4040
Essential oils, herbs

Lavender Lane
7337 #1 Roseville Rd.
Sacramento, CA 95842
(888) 593-4400 or (916) 334-4400
fax: (916) 339-0842
e-mail: donna@lavenderlane.com
website: www.lavenderlane.com
Base oils, bottles and jars, herbs

Mountain Rose Herbs
20818 High St.
North San Juan, CA 95960
(800) 879-3337 or (530) 292-9138
fax: (530) 292-9138
Aloe vera gel, base and essential oils, beeswax, bottles and jars, clays, cocoa butter, floral waters, funnels, glycerin, herbs, labeling supplies, witch hazel

Oak Ridge Farms, Inc.
P.O. Box 28
Basking Ridge, New Jersey 07920
(800) 444-8843
fax: (908) 953-9070
e-mail: oakrigd@ix.netcom.com
website: www.oakridgefarms.com
Herbs

Original Swiss Aromatics
602 Frietas Pkwy.
San Rafael. CA 94903
(415) 479-9121
fax: (415) 479-0119
Absolutes, essential oils

Penn Herb Co.
10601 Decatur Rd.. Ste. 2
Philadelphia. PA 19154
(215) 632-6100
Herbs and herbal extracts

Rabbit Shadow Farm
2880 East Highway 402
Loveland. CO 80537
(303) 667-5531
website: www.frii.com
Herbs

Redmond Minerals, Inc.
P.O. Box 219
Redmond. UT 84652
(800) 367-7258 or (435) 529-7402
fax: (435) 529-7486
Bath salts

SKS Bottle & Packaging Inc.
3 Knabner Rd.
Mechanicsville, NY 12118
(800) 810-0440 or (518) 899-7488
Bottles and jars, labeling supplies

Snowcap
2271 Vauxhall Pl.
Richmond. BC V6V 1Z5
Canada
(800) 561-2868 or (604) 278-4870
Base oils

St. John's Herb Garden, Inc.
7711 Hillmeade Rd.
Bowie. MD 20720
(301) 262-5302
fax: (301) 262-2489
Bottles and jars, herbs, labeling
supplies

Sunburst Bottle Company
5710 Auburn Blvd.. Ste. 7
Sacramento. CA 95841
(916) 348-5576
fax: (916) 348-3808
Bottles and jars, droppers, labeling
supplies, pumps, vials

Wild Weeds
1302 Camp Weott Rd.
Ferndale. CA 95536
(707) 786-4906
website: www.wildweeds.com
Base oils, glass containers, herbs

Organizations

American Botanical Council
P.O. Box 3268
Santa Monica, CA 90408
(800) 437-2362
e-mail: abc@herbalgram.org

**American Herbal Products
Association**
8484 Georgia Ave.. Ste. 370
Silver Springs, MD 20910
(301) 588-1171
fax: (301) 588-1174
e-mail: AHPA@ix.netcom.com

American Herbalist Guild
P.O. Box 70
Roosevelt. UT 84066
(435) 722-8434
fax: (435) 722-8452
e-mail: ahgoffice@earthlink.net
website: www.healthy.net/pan/pa/
herbalmedicine/ahg/index.html

Herb Research Foundation
1007 Pearl St.. Ste. 200
Boulder, CO 80302
(303) 449-2265
fax: (303) 449-7849
e-mail: info@herbs.org
website: www.healthy.net/herbalists

**National Association for Holistic
Aromatheraphy**
836 Hanley Industrial Court
Saint Louis, MO 63144
(888) 275-6242
fax: (314) 963-4454
e-mail: info@naha.org

Publications

American Herb Association
P.O. Box 1673
Nevada City. CA 95959
(530) 265-9552

The Herb Companion
P.O. Box 7714
Red Oak. IA 51591
(800) 456-5835
website: www.Interweave.com

Herb Gathering
10949 East 200
South Lafayette, IN 47905
(765) 296-4116

The Herb Quarterly
Long Mountain Press. Inc.
P.O. Box 689
San Anselmo. CA 94960

HerbalGram
P.O. Box 144345
Austin. TX 78714-4345
(800) 373-7105 or (512) 926-4900
e-mail: custserv@herbalgram.org

Herbs for Health
P.O. Box 7714
Red Oak. IA 51591-0708
(800) 456-6018
website: www.Interweave.com

Herbs & Spices for Home Use
1010 46th St.
Emeryville, CA 94608
(510) 601-0700
fax: (510) 601-0726

Websites

**American Herbal
Pharmacopoeia™**
www.herbal-alp.org

**American Natural Hygiene
Society**
www2.anhs.org/anhs

Flora of North America Project
www.fna.org/index.html

Henrietta's Medicinal Herb FAQ
www.sunsite.unc.edu/herbmed/
mediherb.html

**Herbnet: Herb Growing &
Marketing**
www.herbnet.com

**Index of Herbal/Alternative
Healthcare Databases**
www.sunsite.unc.edu/pub/academic/
medicine/alternative-healthcare

**International Internet Directory
for Botany**
www.herb.biol.uregina.ca/liu/bio/
botany

Index

About the Authors

After fifteen years as a professional chef, **Mike Hulbert** abandoned the restaurant business and moved to the Appalachian Mountains in search of a healthier lifestyle. There he began cultivating and selling herbs, and met and married herbalist **Anna Carter**. Together they have turned Anna's small soap-making company into Creation Herbal Products, a thriving business that supplies natural beauty aids and remedies to anyone seeking nontoxic alternatives to commercially manufactured skin, hair, and medicinal products. Mike Hulbert is the author of COUNTRY LIVING HANDMADE SOAP: RECIPES FOR CRAFTING SOAP AT HOME.

Photo Credits

Photonica: Box Office 30, 86; Tulla Booth 47; Peter Davidian cover (top right), 14, 27; Gentl & Hyers 34, 65, 71, 77, 82, 91, 120; Craig Harris 126; Shinzo Hirai i, vii, ix, x, 69, 109; Mikami (Ima) Kaori cover (bottom left), 67; The Picture Book 60, 104; Erik Rank 25; Deborah Raven 21; Joanne Schmaltz cover (top left), ii; Iwakiri Takashi 115; Yoshinori Uwabo cover (bottom right); Peter Zeray 45

Envision: Steven Mark Needham 75, 103; Andre Baranowsky 119

Gentl & Hyers: v, 17, 40, 51, 54, 57, 95, 98, 110, 128

Acknowledgments

First and foremost, we thank the Lord for making our life and work so meaningful. Special thanks go to Dr. Larry Young and Reverends Ben Cox, Jim Fletcher, and David Long for guiding us along the path; to the past and present members of the North Carolina Herb Association and our local community for supporting our endeavors this past decade; and to our mothers, fathers, and the whole extended family—both biological and spiritual—who believed in our research and helped us prove that herbs really work by allowing us to test our recipes on them—with great results!

We are grateful to Camilla Crichton, Gretchen Mergenthaler, Debbie Sfetsios, and Alanna Stang for tackling the editorial and design complexities of this material with so much patience and good spirits. And to the many people have contributed to this book in countless ways over the last decade, including Lou and Barbara Applebaum, Vicki Baker, Buzz Beeson, Monty and Barbara Carrier, Jerry and Laura Clemmons, J. B. and Pam Coates, Wilma Cooke, Dr. Jeanine Davis, Mary Embler, Bill Glen, Ben Henderson and Mary Underwood, Marylou Johnson, Ron and Dorothy Lee, Tamara Leonard, David Massey, Bobbie Moore, Rick and Jane Morgan, Diane Morris, Alan Salmon and Betty Sparrow, Meg Shelton, Ray and Mary Snead, Tom and Shirley Speight, Cheryl Stippich, Sylvia Tippett, Wayne and Sharon Underwood, Dick and Diane Weaver, Joe and Barbara Weddington.